Bad Theology in a Time of COVID

"With an accessible and confident style, Leah Robinson invites readers to learn and remember amid the ravages of the COVID-19 pandemic. She deftly takes us through Christian theological responses to widespread disease, from The Plague of Justinian to the HIV/AIDS epidemic. For pastors and parishes who care for all kinds of sick folk, for chaplains and healthcare professionals who practice their healing arts every day, and for scholars and students who wrestle with the practical implications of our deepest theological convictions, this is a must read!."

—Thomas Hermans-Webster, *Affiliate Faculty in Methodist and Wesleyan Studies, Memphis Theological Seminary*

"Leah Robinson has written a highly readable, important book in her *Bad Theology* series. While anchored to impressive historical research, her work takes a needed look at the ways bad theology, or in fact a lack of thoughtful theology, has led to present-day divisions and harmful actions on the part of many churches during the COVID pandemic. While the scholarship is clear and evident, I find the true strength of this book to be the heart of Robinson's desire to aid her community in self-reflection and development of theology that is directed toward imitating God and maintaining God's desire for human flourishing. Her love for people motivates her critiques of bad actions, and so the book is not only providing information, but a call to better theology and application of it."

—Kristine Whaley, PhD., *Assistant Professor of Religion and Humanities, St Petersburg College*

"This timely book comes to us at an important moment as we begin to reflect on the causes and consequences of the COVID-19 pandemic. Building upon her excellent *Bad Theology*, Leah Robinson invites us to remember that theology is not contained in our church pews and Bible studies, it is embodied in our communities and the public sphere. This book reminds us that our theological ideas are not private, they impact the world and the people around us."

—Bryant Burkhart, *Drew University, USA*

Leah Robinson

Bad Theology in a Time of COVID

palgrave
macmillan

Leah Robinson
Charlotte, NC, USA

ISBN 978-3-031-75293-3 ISBN 978-3-031-75294-0 (eBook)
https://doi.org/10.1007/978-3-031-75294-0

This Palgrave Macmillan imprint is published by the registered company Springer Nature Switzerland AG.
The registered company address is: Gewerbestrasse 11, 6330 Cham, Switzerland

This book is dedicated to my grandmother, Jerri VZ Robinson.
May you rest in peace and rise in glory.
Love, the girl with the moon pie eyes.

Varys:	Power is a curious thing, my Lord. Are you fond of riddles?
Tyrion:	Why? Am I about to hear one?
Varys:	Three great men sit in a room. A king, a priest, and a rich man. Between them stands a common Sellsword. Each great man bids the Sellsword kill the other two. Who lives? Who dies?
Tyrion:	Depends on the Sellsword.
Varys:	Does it? He has neither crown, nor gold, nor favor with the gods.
Tyrion:	He has a sword-the power of life and death.
Varys:	But if its swordsman who rule, why do we pretend kings hold all the power? When Ned Stark lost his head, who was truly responsible: Joffrey, the executioner, or something else?
Tyrion:	I've decided I don't like riddles.
Varys:	Power resides where men believe it resides. It's a trick. A shadow on the wall. And a very small man can cast a very large shadow.

Varys' Riddle, *Game of Thrones*, HBO

Contents

CHAPTER 1

Prologue

> Michel's death marked, one might say, the end of the first period, that of bewildering portents, and the beginning of another, relatively more trying, in which the perplexity of the early days gradually gave place to panic.[1]

A paper given at "TheoCon" 2020 (virtually)

It seems like only yesterday that I was giving a plenary talk to your LGBTQIA Student Alliance at the University of Edinburgh in February of this year. In just a month's time after that talk, the whole world would be forever different. But we did not know that then. I'm not sure I had one conversation about the virus during that trip; it was all handshakes and hugs, laughter and the breaking of bread. A few weeks later, I headed back over the ocean to Northern Ireland, to lead a trip on peacebuilding and reconciliation with a group of students from Queens University, Charlotte. We used handwipes, and we washed our plane seats down, but we did all the touristy stuff.

And then we returned home, and the slow march of time towards the end of the semester was brought to a screeching halt. And those dinners and drinks in Edinburgh, and my gatherings of planning meetings for Northern Ireland, seem years past. Those of you who know me personally know that I am hardly someone who admits defeat, if ever. I blame it on the years of playing high school sports and supporting the Atlanta Falcons,

[1] Albert Camus, *The Plague* (Vintage International: New York, 1991, 3rd edition), 23.

L. Robinson, *Bad Theology in a Time of COVID*,
https://doi.org/10.1007/978-3-031-75294-0_1

the Georgia Bulldogs, and the Atlanta Braves, who break my heart on a regular basis. However, in this current crisis, and indeed as protests are raging in my home state of Georgia and my adopted city of Charlotte, I feel ever so slightly defeated.

Even as I sat down to write this paper, I could feel the quarantine fatigue setting in. I blamed it on the fact that this was due on the same day as a million-dollar Lily grant that I was putting forward, or the fact my cats were waking me up at 5 a.m. every morning for some reason, or the fact that until now I had no desk because I had to give my desk to my IT husband who apparently needs six monitors in order to do his job, and so I tried to convince myself I was Truman Capote and would write my great works from my bed.

But in all honesty, the fatigue is really the quarantine, and being left with our own thoughts. It's not having time demarcated- it's days fading into nights and weeks into months. It's missing family and friends and missing the framework that sets our lives and our mental health into a rhythm that is pleasing. And as a practical theologian, I'd be amiss not to say if you are struggling with this virus, the isolation, the sickness, and even the death, I hear you. Or if you are mourning the racism that exists in your home country, I see you. Or you feel like the leadership you are forced to follow does not speak for you, I'm giving you a virtual hug. You are not alone, and my prayer is that this conference offers you some sense of structure. Perhaps it offers some sense of relief, or in this case, a sense of calling to justice. We are all with you, trust me. The weariness of this time is a real thing, and so I'm very grateful to you for being here.

If any of you have heard me speak before, you know that I am unashamedly an evangelist in my love for being a practical theologian. It's probably my lone evangelical quality, honestly. So, it was an honor and a delight to be given the practical theological section of this particular conference. And as I'm of the strong belief that all theology is practical, it made sense in the context. So please allow me to offer you my academic Tinder profile speech. Hi, Friend or Stranger! My name is Rev. Dr. Leah E. Robinson. I was born and raised in a town called Ringgold, Georgia. I was raised in the church, the Southern Baptist Church, to be specific. I went to school for religion in undergraduate and then on to seminary at Mercer University in Atlanta. I'm an ordained minister in the Christian Church (Disciples of Christ). I studied for my PhD in Practical Theology at the University of Edinburgh. The subject of my PhD was the theology of reconciliation, as told through the lens of people from Northern Ireland. I previously worked at the University of Glasgow as a University Teacher in Practical Theology and Peacebuilding, the University of Edinburgh as Lecturer in Practical and Pastoral Theology, and Pfeiffer University as Associate Professor of Religion. I have served as a minister, a youth minister, a chaplain, and a university professor in both the UK and the USA now for 14 years. I have published in journals that range from *Practical Theology* to the *Victorian Review* and offered chapters on subjects that range from sectarianism in Scottish sports to feminist trauma theology. My first book *Embodied Peacebuilding: Reconciliation as Practical Theology* is out now. My newest book, which we will be talking a lot about today, is entitled *Bad Theology: Oppression in the Name of God* and it is out with SCM Press.

I thought of all the many ways that I could present my paper today. Practical theology has, in the USA, been associated with ministerial studies, but we know in the academy that practical theology goes far beyond that. It encompasses all theology. It is theology in the world. The arms and legs of theology. Embodied theology, but that term can have its own issues related to inclusivity. So, my definition for this paper is, because when I look in my mind's eye for even a moment all I can see is George Floyd's picture, I am going to say that practical theology is theology that is breathed. For as long as we have the privilege of breath, practical theology is incarnated in this world. Whether that is spoken word, written word, or theology embodied. The reality of describing practical theology that way is the sheer scope of the subject at hand. Practical theology is a big umbrella of theological discussions, so I could have looked at many different ways that theology interplays with human life in a pandemic such as health, science, tech, politics, the public sphere, worship (and now online worship), and so on.

But instead, I chose to follow my research. I have for many years been wrestling with the idea of naming theology that is oppressive or damaging as bad theology. I was scared to do that at first because it comes with so many debates about criteria and conclusions and definitions of bad and good which are so subjective. So, I put it on the shelf for a while. But in the past few years, it has come down again. And as I contemplated how I was going to frame this paper, the following news story popped up into my feed from a minister named Rev. William H. Lamar IV, pastor of the Metropolitan African Methodist Episcopal Church in Washington DC. The Op-Ed read, "William H. Lamar IV-it's not just the Coronavirus,

Bad Theology is killing us."[2] I will go into what Lamar says about all of this, but before even reading it I realized how brave it was to name your article in such a way. Lamar was naming something that he saw as an injustice. He was using his breath to speak out against a named enemy of his community. He was brave. And while one person's bad theology is another person's good theology—depending on your community and perspective—I believe there is still merit in naming and discussing these perspectives in order to see where hurt is taking place in the name of God. And so now in 2020, I am going to start a conversation about bad theology in a time of Coronavirus. I say start because this paper is not a five-point thesis and conclusion. This paper is the start of a conversation that should result in debate and discussion. Some people will agree and others will not, and that is absolutely the way that theology should be. Until someone gets God's cell phone, these debates should ever be. And why do I do this? Why write this paper and this book? Although I'm not one to drop Bible verses into academic papers, the why in these questions relates to the following Bible verse. Matthew 10:16 (NRSV) "See I am sending you out like sheep into the midst of wolves; so be as wise as serpents and innocent as doves."

The imagery is profound if examined closely. We are being called to be two seemingly opposing images in this sentence. On the one hand, the innocence of the dove, who is seen as a worthy sacrifice to God. On the other hand, the imagery of the snake, one associated with deceit, deception, and cunningness. We are supposed to be operating in both of those spheres at once. But why? Why must we be innocent in God's eyes, yet wise as serpents?

Because we live in a broken beat-up world. And Jesus knew that. And this is why I am looking at bad theology. If you are Christian, it is oftentimes easy to fall into the routine of hearing anyone who speaks for your corner of Christianity as being right or true or good. But this is perilous. No matter what side of the theological world you reside. We are called to be innocent, faithful, and loyal, but we are also called to discern, to name,

[2] William H. Lamar IV, "It's not just the coronavirus-bad theology is killing us," *Faith And Leadership* https://faithandleadership.com/william-h-lamar-iv-its-not-just-the-coronavirus-bad-theology-killing-us [accessed 2/8/24].

and to discuss. Because not all theology that is out there is beneficial. And while I'm not pretentious enough to say what is absolutely good and bad theology, I, like, William Lamar IV, see the benefit of starting a conversation of naming bad theology and seeing where it goes.

Edinburgh University, 2020

CHAPTER 2

Introduction

> In fact, like our fellow citizens, Rieux was caught off his guard, and we should understand his hesitations in the light of this fact and similarly understand how he was torn between conflicting fears and confidence. When a war breaks out, people say: "If it's too stupid; it can't last long." But though a war may well be "too stupid," that doesn't prevent its lasting. Stupidity has a knack of getting its way; as we should see if we were not always so much wrapped up in ourselves.[1]

In March 2020, I had the privilege of taking students from Queens University, Charlotte to my beloved Northern Ireland. We had heard whispers and mumblings of the virus at this stage, but no cases in the USA had been reported. My mother warned me that she had heard of a case in Dublin, and there was cause for some concern. On this trip, I was able to show students the country that I researched for my PhD. We washed our hands and sanitized our seats, but no one was too concerned. As I showed the students the places we had discussed in books, and as we sat and had conversations, difficult conversations, about all we were learning, I felt so delighted that the theories and stories that I had written about in my PhD were coming to life in a new generation. A new generation that would wrestle with global issues in a way that I could not have imagined as an

[1] Camus, *The Plague*, 37.

L. Robinson, *Bad Theology in a Time of COVID*,
https://doi.org/10.1007/978-3-031-75294-0_2

elder millennial with dial-up internet. That trip was one of the best moments of my academic career.

Then, on March 25, 2020, I was on a podcast with my colleague, friend, and fellow theologian Kevin Taylor. Lockdown in the United States had just begun, and I was lamenting to him on our podcast *Theology is Annoying* that my hairdresser had said she might be out of work for three whole weeks because of the pandemic. She was disappointed and worried, and I was shocked. Later, Kevin told me that he thought that I was being dramatic during that conversation about how long she would be unable to return to her salon. That was the beginning, and how little we knew about what was to come.

By the summer of 2020, we all knew that this was not something that was going away anytime soon. We were bombarded with information, sometimes conflicting, and we were trying to navigate a new world that was full of invisible bad guys at every corner. People were getting sick. Loved ones were dying from the virus. Each day I would get on the internet to see the number of those infected and dead tick, quickly, upwards. It was at this time that my friends and former colleagues, Sarah Lane Ritchie and Tripp Fuller, decided to create a conference in the midst of the pandemic. The one thing you can depend on with us theology nerds is that any major event that happens in the world will quickly become the source of a conference in a short amount of time. TheoCon was born out of the minds of these two scholars as well as in the midst of the global pandemic. It was June 2020, and so we had some reflection, but we were truly still battling the war at this stage. I was asked to speak, and the section in the prologue seemed an appropriate way to reflect on where I was during that time, but also, to introduce myself to readers of this text.

When I looked online for articles about the COVID-19 pandemic and theology in July 2020, the results were slim. Not even theologians have that quick of a turnaround in terms of books and articles. One article that stuck out to me was from the Rev. William Lamar IV that I mentioned in the prologue. One of the reasons the article was especially appealing to click was because of the title of the article "bad theology is killing us." The book I was writing at the time was titled, *Bad Theology: Oppression in the Name of God*,[2] so as soon as I saw that article, I was intrigued. It framed my entire talk at TheoCon because it was the first time in the COVID era that I had heard someone speak about the pandemic's influence on

[2] Leah Robinson, *Bad Theology: Oppression in the Name of God* (SCM Press: London, 2023).

theological conclusions and consequences. It will also frame this book in many ways.

In the article, Lamar says that he is doing investigations looking for "theological fingerprints"[3] of those who have hurt his congregation (and congregations of color generally as well as poor white communities). The hurt he speaks of is the imbalance between the COVID deaths of people of color and middle/upper-class white people. He speaks specifically about the numbers of those who died in the USA at this early stage of the pandemic. There has been extensive work done on this topic on the CDC website[4] as well as "The Color of Coronavirus" website.[5]

While the numbers are interesting to look at and scrutinize, my interest in the article reached a peak when Lamar began to speak about the theological reasons that he saw for his community struggling during the pandemic. Simply put, Lamar says that politics needs a theological system to keep it in power. And, consequently, at the heart of the pandemic, Lamar believes, there is politics. He says: "What kind of God-talk makes possible a refusal to provide the universal health care that may have mitigated this crisis? What kind of God-talk makes possible a refusal to invest the money necessary to end homelessness? What kind of God-talk makes possible the racializing of criminality and poverty? What kind of God-talk gives political power to science-denying policymakers? The answer? White evangelical God-talk. The injustices that many communities are experiencing as a result of the novel coronavirus are inextricably linked to this theology."[6] While I do have some contrary thoughts with some of the labels in this quote, the thought of theology being at the root of deaths in the pandemic was of interest to me and my research in bad theology. Lamar goes on to characterize his understanding of "white, evangelical" theology and how it works with governmental entities in order to maintain colonialistic control over the USA. This theology, according to Lamar, is more about keeping the status quo than saving souls, or in this case saving lives from a pandemic.

It is a strong statement to be sure, but it reads as a pastor who is frustrated with the way that his congregation is being failed by the structures

[3] Lamar, "It's not just the coronavirus-bad theology is killing us."

[4] Center of Disease Control, https://www.cdc.gov/nchs/covid19/mortality-overview.htm [accessed 2/8/24].

[5] Color of Coronavirus, https://www.apmresearchlab.org/covid/deaths-by-race [accessed 2/8/24].

[6] Lamar, "It's not just the coronavirus-bad theology is killing us."

that are supposed to be supportive. He concludes his article with the following about those who are being failed by the government in the pandemic: "They cannot socially distance in tight, squalid quarters. They cannot wash their hands in lead-ridden water in Flint. We are having digital funerals for people who live in a city where Congress refuses to extend the health benefits that they themselves enjoy. This bad theology of who belongs and who does not, of who is worthy and who is not, has the blood of my parishioners on its hands."[7]

I was challenged deeply by this article at this point in the pandemic. So, I began searching for specifics when it comes to this "evangelical" theology that Lamar spoke. I am a practical theologian, so I like being able to see things in embodied form in order to talk about them fully. Using Lamar's article as a starting point meant that I was able to look further into where theology was being used to maintain power, to limit human flourishing, and ultimately cause death. One of the beautiful aspects of theology is the privilege of being able to interpret the words of Jesus. Also, to see how they have been interpreted throughout history. It is what made me fall in love with theology in the first place. The dark side of this particular realm of interpretation is when theology is/has been used as a means of justification for evils of unimaginable measure.

In *Bad Theology*, I make it clear that I do not think it is possible for personal bias to not influence theology. We are humans doing a human activity (we will revisit all this in Chap. 1). That being said, is it possible to look at the COVID-19 crisis and be able to point to specific examples where theology hindered instead of helped? Where it was the source of malice and not joy? Where it did not encourage thriving but instead instigated suffering? Did bad theology aid in the staggering death toll that we see in the USA, currently over a million people?[8] I believe so.

The first chapter of this book will revisit my views on Bad Theology because I will throw that phrase around and it bears a reminder of what I have written previously in this regard. I will say that *Bad Theology* has been criticized at points for being too theory-heavy, despite my examples in the second half (i.e., reads like two different books), but I stand by this decision. If you want to dig deep into the way that I came up with a very contentious idea like bad theology, then please go back and read that

[7] Lamar, "It's not just the coronavirus-bad theology is killing us."

[8] Center of Disease Control, https://covid.cdc.gov/covid-data-tracker/#datatracker-home [accessed 2/8/24].

book, so you can see my theology degree at work. For this work, I will assume you know how I came up with the criteria and will focus more on the practical conclusions of that text.

In Chap. 2, I offer a history of the way pandemics have been viewed, theologically speaking. One thing I have learned about teaching history is that humans forget very easily. That is not to say that they can't remember, but they need reminding. When I read about historic pandemics and how theology was used in them for ill or goodwill, I was painfully reminded of our own situation. I sat with Albert Camus, recalling his fictional tales of a pandemic in France in the 1900s, and winced at how similar the reactions in the story were to the ones that I saw in the USA during our own version. The phrase, if you do not learn history you will be forced to repeat it, is true in my mind. Camus called our responses to COVID-19 down to a T in his book, and it was published in 1948.

So what was the perfect storm that meant that the USA sounded like a sequel to a Camus novel? People have blamed many areas of American life that meant that we handled the pandemic way worse than many other developed nations. I have contemplated this in my own writings. Academics will oftentimes see the world through the lens of the subject that they research, as though the whole of the world revolves around xyz. I'm not sure anyone who immerses themselves so fully in very specific subjects as we do can get around that, as annoying as it may be (especially to our loved ones, sorry Stu). I am no exception to this academic pitfall. I see the word in theology, and how it is practiced in the world. As a result, the third chapter will discuss prosperity, premillenialism, politics, and partisanship. I go so far as to say that I hold that these are the reasons that the pandemic was so bad in the USA. That if these theological concepts were not so firmly engrained in the very fabric of the American way of life, then the pandemic may not have been so devastating. I will argue that these four concepts were the foundation of bad theology during COVID-19.

The fourth and fifth chapters are deeply connected. I will always lead my dear readers from theory to practice, typical practical theologian behavior. I have a long list of church leaders and TV evangelists who are on the theological naughty list in light of the pandemic. Those who were COVID-19 deniers, while the numbers climbed, to those who sold healing products on TV to fearful Americans. These people, these ministers, misguided people into putting themselves into dangerous scenarios: physically, spiritually, mentally, and financially.

Finally, we will talk about what we learned. The beauty of practical theology is that we do not like writing for writing's sake. Theory alone is not going to get us out of bed. Not everything has to be wrapped up in a nice bow, but there is a desire to reflect on what we can take away from all that we have lived and theologized through. I could have ended this book with a section on good theology during the pandemic, and I encourage you to look to the ministers who stood up for their congregations. These ministers, like Lamar, attempted to offer some light in the midst of the fog. Good theology is not the conclusion of this story, though. By highlighting the bad theology in the midst of COVID-19, we are talking about what is now history. Remember what I said about history and repeating it. I would challenge that in order to not repeat it we must hold these folks accountable for what they did. We must do this before they fall into the annals of forgetfulness, which is, arguably, a place that is comforting for many of us to put aspects of this terrible time period.

A final word that I offered while doing bad theology: It is ok if you do not agree with my conclusions. An unfortunate hangover from the peak of COVID-19 is that it seems we have lost the ability to have conversations with each other. Even if they are about the most mundane of things. They are now culture-war fodder. I am writing a book on COVID-19 and God. Two topics that inevitably will lead to division in thoughts. I want to affirm that that is exactly the intention and there is nothing wrong with taking a pause. I took pause with some things that I read about COVID-19 and honestly, I was outright confused at others (raises fist at the CDC and all its information!). Disagreeing, with love and respect, is a skill that I teach in my classroom, and one that I always use when writing my books (for the most part). Just because the information does not fit our worldview, or does not align exactly with what we think, does not mean we should not read it in order to expand (or confirm) our own thinking. So, with that being said, stop banning books, and let us get started.

CHAPTER 3

Bad Theology Revisited

> At first, the fact of being cut off from the outside world was accepted with more or less good grace, much as people would have put up with any other temporary inconvenience that interfered with only a few of their habits. But now they had abruptly become aware that they were undergoing a sort of incarceration under that blue dome of sky; already beginning to sizzle in the fires of summer, they had a vague sensation that their whole lives were threatened by the present turn of events, and in the evening, when the cooler air revived their energy, this feeling of being locked in like criminals prompted them sometimes to foolhardy acts.[1]

> For now we see only a reflection, as in a mirror, but then we will see face to face. Now I know only in part; then I will know fully, even as I have been fully known.[2]

It seems like a million years ago that I wrote *Bad Theology: Oppression in the Name of God*. Not because, like the plague in Camus' book, one might wish to push down traumatic events from memory, but because so much has happened in our world since I first envisioned creating this text. As has been mentioned previously, the inspiration for the text came in

[1] Camus, *The Plague*, 100.
[2] 1 Corinthians 13:12, New Revised Standard Updated Version, Bible Gateway https://www.biblegateway.com/passage/?search=1+Corinthians+13%3A12&version=NRSVUE [accessed 4/6/24].

L. Robinson, *Bad Theology in a Time of COVID*,
https://doi.org/10.1007/978-3-031-75294-0_3

2009, in the days of my PhD. Unlike any other text that I've written, the ideas were allowed to be planted, watered, and flourish in my mind. As I finished my PhD, started teaching, wrote up research projects, and moved to the USA to teach again, they grew. As I read texts for teaching, or interacted with groups for research, I subconsciously was collecting information that would later provide the theoretical framework for my understanding of Bad Theology.

Bad Theology is a tale of two halves. The first half being the heavy lifting theologically. This is the spot where I lay out my arguments, systematic theology style, in defense of how I define bad theology. One review said it read like two books, which I absolutely agree with. For those who have not read the book, while the first half is theory (as mentioned), the second half offers practical examples of bad theology throughout history. Some people preferred the theory, and many others preferred the examples, and that is to be expected depending on what side of theology one resides. All that to say, I contend that it was absolutely necessary to have both sides of this book. I could not have argued one without the other. Who am I to say a theological stance is "bad" if not to have support from other theologians upon whose ideas I built my thoughts? That being said, who am I to put forth a theoretical framework without testing it in the real world? The historical nature of the examples were on purpose, as I eased myself into this world of declaring something as bad theology. I was also careful with the scenarios I chose to use as examples. Circumstances in history that most people would agree were negative in nature is a relatively easy way to defend a theory on bad theology. One reviewer said that it would be far harder to recreate this exercise in situations that were current, and I agree. This text is different than the previous in that sense, as it looks to say events that are still happening around us are, in fact, bad theology. All this to say, in order to save you a bit of reading time, I will summarize some of my ideas about bad theology to give you your own guide as we move through current examples. It will be like a cheat sheet of the previous book, and I will be interested to see if you agree as you read along. A final warning and an invitation before we begin. This is a summary of my previous theories, so in order to see the full courtroom defense, please pick up and read *Bad Theology: Oppression in the Name of God*. You're welcome, SCM Press.

An aspect of my own journey as a theologian is that I self-identify as a practical theologian. Those who are reading this text that are not in the day-to-day dreary arguments about what constitutes systematic theology, historical theology, dogmatic theology, or practical theology will maybe not be as interested in this stance. That makes complete sense to someone who is an academic in one world and a minister in another. The main thing within these arguments about theology (chats about God) is that much like everything else in this world, there are debates about the best way to go about things. Practical theologians typically discuss theology in terms of beliefs, actions, rituals, trends, and so on that they can see in the world. As a result, their theological conclusions are often constructions of what they have empirically observed around them. This is not always the case, of course, but it is a key level of distinction in regard to more abstract or philosophical musings about the nature of God. Practical theologians rarely claim to know God's actions and intentions in the world, but we do claim to know what people are doing in the world. The interpretations of God's actions and intentions through the human condition say a lot about humans and a lot about God, many Practical Theologians contend. Don Browning takes the position that all theology is practical in nature (i.e., only observable from its human projections). Any theology that claims to be theoretical or philosophical was once observable theology that has been abstracted into a consumable system. There is nothing wrong with this type of systematic understanding of theology, but he is very quick to say that we cannot take this as objective truth about God because of the origins of these theological systems being based on human understanding. He argues that we can learn a lot about how much of our "dogmatic" or "denominational" theology that we take as fact was first seen being enacted in communities. This stance as the theological framework behind *Bad Theology* is made apparent throughout my original text. It is foundational because it states that theology comes from somewhere. It is a construction of the human variety. Is it also a heavenly gift, bestowed upon a precious few? Perhaps. But I contend that there are people who claim this heavenly inspiration who could maybe use further review, and it is for this reason that I wrote *Bad Theology*.

Many would ask, what about the Holy Spirit? How do we know what is really from God when we analyze humans? My answer is that we do not know. This was really the basis for bad and good theology (and their criteria). Gordon Kaufman, someone I use often in my original text, has a useful understanding of this issue in theological studies. Kaufman is quoted in *Bad Theology* as saying: "Theology is human work. Theology is done by humans for human purposes; theological work must be assessed by human standards, and its judges are themselves always ordinary humans."[3] This does not mean that there is no divine inspiration, which I want to highlight again, but what it does mean is that we may need to discern some of these theological conclusions in light of the reality of their inspiration. Kaufman discusses the idea of "God" and "Reality God." Kaufman argues that it is difficult, if not impossible, to know the entirety of Reality God-as God is. This is simply because we are humans and not God. That being said, we have a concept of God in the sense that we are operating in communities of worship and devotion. We have the Holy Spirit and we have the teachings of Jesus. But, even with these guides, there are contradictions and differences in the Christian church. This reality means that either one group is absolutely correct and the others are wrong (which is a commonly held belief between some Christian denominations) or the other option is that everyone has a piece of the absolute correct nature of God. We may just not have the complete picture because of the influence of our social context and our limited ability to comprehend, completely, otherworldly ideas.

What I want to reiterate here is that this is not a reason to despair. If anything, it could be a concept that brings Christians together as a questioning and discerning community of faith, which at the core, is what faith is. However, historically, this has meant feuding and warring between members of the same overarching group of Christians. We put our flags in the sand and we jump in our trenches against those of our same tradition. Ultimately, I would argue, this reflects human desire to have a firm foundation in what is objective and true and consequently what is not. It is a tall order for any discipline, let alone a discipline that involves a seemingly unmeasurable source of knowledge. But when it comes to life and death, it is where we find ourselves.

With all of this as a background, we move now to the criteria themselves. If, at a baseline, we accept that different Christian denominations have different interpretations of the same scripture, we can begin to move towards an understanding that some of these theological conclusions may not be the same as others. Throughout history, we have more or less accepted that different Christian denominations have reached different theological conclusions to similar problems, and to varying degrees. We may not think about it that much, but we are standing alongside our

[3] Gordan Kaufman, *The Theological Imagination* (Philadelphia: Westminster Press, 1981), 263.

Christian brothers and sisters with sometimes diametrically opposed opinions on the same topic. The way that we reconcile this disconnect is that we bury ourselves inside our own denominational echo chamber and try to avoid comparing and contrasting too much. Or, we take our beliefs and bury ourselves in our own denominational echo chamber and say that the other groups are just flat-out wrong. This is also a common theological turn. My focus on bad theology related predominately to the second group. This makes sense since the theological conclusions of these groups are so outrageous that there needed to be self-justification in their actions. The best way to self-justify is to say that you are right and everyone else is wrong, especially in circumstances where self-justification is a tricky endeavor. These were the historical examples that I focused on in the book. These examples ranged from theological justifications of apartheid in South Africa to massacres of native people in the early colonies, to the KKK, to Jonestown. In each example, I showed how a relatively benign systematic idea of theology had been manipulated and used for bad when enacted in a practical way. The theological ideas that I showed had been used for evil in these scenarios were as follows: providence, election, tradition, and eschatology.

As mentioned, these are all relatively neutral terms in the abstract, but in my examples, they took on a life of their own. Providence, a concept that offers the idea that God is looking out for God's people in the world, is not a theology that would create an initial sense of dread. Simply put, God has a plan for the world, humans included, and God is actively working to bring about this plan according to God's will. Again, all very straightforward as it stands, that is, until the idea of providence is used to oppress an entire group of people. Providence can be weaponized in a way where certain groups of people claim that they are acting out God's plan in the world, but in the process, they are oppressing others as a means to an end. In my example, we see this in apartheid-era South Africa. There was a strong us versus them mentality between black South Africans and Europeans who came to occupy the nation. Claiming intimate knowledge of God's plans for South Africa, the Europeans who came to these lands brought a version of Christianity that elevated their own status based on race and religious beliefs. At the same time, they used theology to exclude black people from any conversation involving political power. Even Christian, black people.

This version of a theology of providence assumed a great deal about the purpose of God in South Africa. It was a theology of domination at any cost, even the lives and well-being of fellow humans. It was also a theology of exclusion for the sake of the chosen community of Europeans. The world of South Africa was separated at every turn, whether that was education, entertainment, or even transportation (to name a few). This was seen as being theologically justified because the European colonists had a relationship with God that was special. They were the bearers of the good news, and they were the ones who had been chosen to come to this land and convert those they met. It is a real question as to how one converts people they do not interact with on a daily basis, but that did not seem to concern folks too much in this world.

I have to be transparent since I began to study election in my seminary career, I found it a difficult concept. There is something about setting aside a group of people as being "special" in God's eyes that appeared automatically problematic. This is maybe because I did not grow up in a Calvinist church, or that I did grow up in a divided Deep South, but either way, when it was presented to me as a historical, theological concept, I had questions. Election, at its core, is the idea that God is all-powerful and operates how God wants to operate in the world. This includes electing for certain things to happen at a given time. To follow the logic of election, this also means that God has knowledge about events prior to them happening. Israel is God's chosen people in the Hebrew texts, and this is no accident according to those who are proponents of election. God knew, has known, and will know the people that are faithful to God-self.

But the question remains: Who are God's chosen people outside of what is stated in the text? This is the rub. If a group states that they are an elected group of people, it is difficult to combat that (unless you use some bad theology criteria). This is exactly what happened with the Puritans as they made their way to the North American colonies. The Puritans were a group of Protestants who felt as though the newly created Church of England (Anglican) needed further reforms in order to be the church it was supposed to be. Needless to say, England took issue with these calls for reforms, seeing them as subversion to the crown itself. The Puritans were humored for a while by the monarchy, but they soon realized they were being marginalized because of their views on the future of the church in England. The colonies in North America represented a new start for the Puritans. A place where they could create their utopian society that was based on their own values and their own understandings. England was happy enough to see them go and granted them areas within the Massachusetts Bay Colony to reside. More and more Puritans left England for the colonies as they were convinced they were being called as a chosen people to a chosen land. A land, as we see in the Hebrew scriptures, that was just for them.

Manifest destiny is a common theme in election discussions as it relates to colonialization. The idea is that a group of people are destined to create a new nation in a new world as a chosen people. There are both theological and logistical issues with this concept. For one, the new nations are rarely new and are usually occupied by entire nations of people who did not get a memo from God about their ousting. Secondly, theologically speaking, there is a feeling with those who feel elected to take over a nation, that they are doing so under the instruction and desire of an all-knowing God. As a result, those who already occupy a land are preventing the elect from following through with God's plan for the country itself. With this us versus them mentality, with God as the hype person for the elect, the people who live in lands that are desired by others become non-persons in the eyes of the elect. If these people decide to convert to the religion of the elect, that is fine, but it is not necessary for the elect's ultimate plan. If they do not convert, and try to fight back, there is nothing that the elect will not do to complete their divinely ordained plan.

Hopefully, at this stage, the issues are clear. When John Winthrop and his group of Puritans were confronted with the indigenous people of North America, they were less than hospitable. Using the doctrine of election, they enacted incredible acts of violence against First Peoples in these early years of the colonies. There were some voices in the colonies that tried to fight against those in charge in order to form a fairer society. People like Roger Williams, who wanted to pay indigenous people for their lands, were quickly exiled for insubordination. Nothing would get in between the Puritans and their election by God to create a shining example of a city on a hill. The consequences of this plan were the deaths of entire groups of native peoples at the hands of those who claimed to be chosen to do God's work in the world.

Who does not love a good tradition? There is something about gathering together a community of people and repeating certain rituals or acts in order to remember your origin stories as a group. Some of these stories might be hard and some of them joyous beyond measure, but tradition means that despite the good or the bad, there is a sense of bonding when people remember the ties that bind them together. But what about when the things that bring us together as a group are used as a means of creating a scenario where there is an in-group and an out-group? This is what happens when theologies around tradition are used to draw a line between insiders and outsiders. Inherently, traditions separate us from one another, but this separation does not necessarily lend itself to violence or oppression. But it can. This is especially true depending on how sharply these lines are drawn between groups. Are we celebrating our connectedness as a group, or are we celebrating our superiority in comparison to people outside the group?

This is the story of a bad theology of tradition in relation to the Ku Klux Klan (KKK). There was always a sense of separation from current history when it comes to the KKK. They embody a mythos that they are both in this world, but at the same time wise beyond this world in terms of their outdated ideologies. To explain this in a practical sense, the first incarnation of the KKK came about in a post-civil war era, wherein men returning from war were confronted with a world that had effectively moved on without them. The freeing of the slaves, especially in the South, marked a triumphant period for the United States. For those who had owned slaves, or lived in a world that had forever had a separation of the races, it marked a period of a loss of a tradition. In this case, tradition is not just a sacred thing, it can also mean a repetition of behaviors and ways of life for certain groups of people. The Civil War marked an end to a tradition of evil that had pervaded society since the beginning of the USA itself. Many celebrated, many did not. Those who did not celebrate chose to fight to maintain their traditions like their salvation depended on it. And for many, this was the belief at the time.

In those early, post-war days, the Klan had a singular focus: "By 1870, there were branches of the KKK in almost every southern state. The first incarnation of the Klan was hyper-focused on reinstating the status quo in the south—that is, white supremacy. So while the KKK's actions were not always coordinated, their goal was clear."[4] The traditions, or repeated behaviors and actions of this group, were essential to the ways of the old south. The new south was moving on to a new reality. The KKK was looking to maintain that which it viewed it had lost. Namely, power. Furthering this desire for a return to the past with a good mixture of religions meant that the KKK created a theological justification for their outdated tradition. It was on this theological foundation that they furthered their cause throughout history.

[4] Leah Robinson, *Bad Theology: Oppression in the Name of God* (London: SCM Press, 2023), 126.

Eschatology as a theological term is central to the message of Jesus. In non-theology terms, it essentially means the study of the end times. Jesus spoke often about his return to earth in the New Testament. Post Gospels, in Revelation alone, there are four lines of scripture that discuss the return coming soon.[5] This was a promise to those in the early church who were devastated and confused by the death/resurrection of Jesus. Leaderless, early Christians needed this promise to keep them going amidst persecution that surrounded them in the Roman Empire. The oppression did not end with Jesus' death and resurrection, and so early followers of Jesus needed something to hold on to.

As the years have passed since that time, Christians continue to cling to this idea that Jesus will return, and return soon. I am convinced that this language of return and soon was not intended for what they would theologically evolve to be in the here and now. With the addition of New Testament interpretations that say there would be terrible times of war and violence before Jesus' return, theologians set up a situation whereby people throughout history have thought that the time of return is now. This is, unfortunately, because humans are never not at war, so the timing seems always to be now or at least soon. In theory, this can create a sense of hope, but it can also set up a situation of divine disappointment.

Alongside disappointment, there is also the danger that dwelling on the end times can be used as a source of manipulation. In *Bad Theology*, I discuss the idea of a bad theology of eschatology in relation to the Jonestown massacre. In this scenario, the pastor Jim Jones convinced a congregation of people to give away their possessions and move to South America to create a utopian society. This could have been the end of the story, but alas it is not. Jonestown quickly became a place of ever-changing theology by Jones, as well as increased paranoia and oppression. Not at all the utopia that had been promised, many members of Jonestown decided to leave. There is probably nothing worse for a cult leader with terrible theology than a loss of disciples. The blow to the ego must have been enormous.

In the end, Jones created a theology that leaned heavily into the end times. He claimed that there were no other options for the group at Jonestown beyond taking their own lives. Jones stated that because of the lifestyle they chose to live, they were going to be persecuted forever by outside forces. As a result, the option that was the best for everyone was to take ownership of their lives by ending them by their own hand. Some

[5] Rev 16:15; 22:7,12,20.

members of the community disagreed and tried to escape, but were not successful because of Jones. The majority, however, agreed to go through with mass suicide via self-poisoning. More than 900 people died that day in South America, including mothers and their children. They were victims of Jones and his bad theology about the end times. The people he claimed were going to be relentless in persecuting the group were, in fact, sent by families of the members to check on them and help them out. To Jones, this was unacceptable, and so he ended the community much like he had started it, based on bad theology, good words, and a sense that the end was soon. The members did not know how true that was going to be.

As I have been going through these examples, I have used the phrase bad theology multiple times. In *Bad Theology*, I spent a great deal of time mapping out my methodology when it came to what I was going to eventually label as good and bad theology. While this process can be tedious, it was also very necessary. It is why I am glad I can summarize it in this text, while still having the full version in my previous text for reference. Because I am firmly in the world of practical theology, it can be a bit jarring for readers of my work to have to go on this long journey of self-justification in my choices. Usually, I am busy constructing theology that others have given me via qualitative research, or I am reading about the embodiment of theology in texts about real-life people. Most people in the world of PT, or students, or people doing ministry in the world, will not necessarily care about pages of theologians throughout history who have agreed with my criteria on good and bad theology. But again, I say that this was too big of a risk to just say a list of theological criteria without using theological friends along the way. I had read too much bad theology whereby people did not have any justification for their conclusions. No theological friends at all. Sometimes you need people to agree with you in order to know that you are not creating something completely erroneous or dangerous.

Now with that being said, the second point that I made in my methodological section was the idea that at some point we are all erroneous (we can be this without being dangerous and I will get to that later). We are erroneous because we are just humans and God is infinite. As a result, we can only understand God in parts and not a complete whole. These parts are oftentimes muddled in our context and our own biases and viewpoints. This again is why it is important to have other theologians who are from different contexts who have said similar things to you, theological friends as I call them. It is not just to say, this person is smart and went to a fancy school and agrees with me so therefore you must also agree. Instead, it is saying all those things, but also that they thought of the idea before me. They worked out this idea in a different time and place, and we are coming to the same conclusions. So while 100% accuracy is not possible in my theological methodology, there is an idea that you can join a cloud of witnesses to try and explain something in our best human way.

A quote that helped underpin a great deal of my methodology of *Bad Theology* comes from the Southern writer Flannery O'Connor: "A God you understood would be less than yourself."[6] At the center of my theological inquiry is the idea that humans are not capable of understanding God as Godself is complete. I am not alone in this thought. Two of my best theological friends in this journey are Gordon Kaufman and Kathryn Tanner.

Kaufman makes the distinction between what he calls reality God and God. Reality God is the true nature of Godself which, as O'Connor stated, is not completely knowable by the finite mind of humans. That being said, humans are able to get bits of God through things like inspiration and the Holy Spirit. These bits are constructed through a human's lens of context, culture, and general views of the world. It is through this construction that we get Kaufman's version of God. God is not reality God, but it is a God that we have constructed as best as we can. Kaufman's ideas about this construction of God mirror other theologians, such as Karl Barth. Although I lean more towards Kaufman's ideas than Barth's, it is worth noting that during an argument with fellow theologian Emil Brunner, Barth also discussed the unknowable God. In this back and forth, Barth states: "The possibility of real knowledge by natural man of the true God, derived from creation is, according to Calvin, a possibility in principle, but not in fact, not a possibility to be realised by us."[7] Brunner believed that humans were capable of knowing the nature of God through the revelation of creation and the natural world. In other words, we are who we are and the world is what it is because we were created by God. This creative element means we have a window into the essence of God. Barth, being ever focused on Jesus above all things, does contend that humans can know about God through the incarnation of Jesus, but even that is

[6] Flannery O'Connor, The Center for Contemplative Practice, https://thecenterforcontemplativepractice.org/2022/02/25/flannery-oconnor-gods-pit-bull/ [accessed 5/6/24].

[7] Karl Barth in Emil Brunner and Karl Barth, *Natural Theology: Comprising 'Nature and Grace' by Professor Dr. Emil Brunner and the reply 'No!' by Dr. Karl Barth*, trans. Peter Fraenkel (Eugene: Wipf and Stock, 2002), 106.

interpreted through a human lens. On this, we can agree. I do believe that reality God can be known through the person of Jesus, but the scriptures were written by humans, and their interpretations (theology) were concluded by humans. As 1 Corinthians 13:12 states: "For now we see only a reflection, as in a mirror, but then we will see face to face. Now I know only in part; then I will know fully, even as I have been fully known."[8]

Another theologian that I use heavily in my methodology section is Kathryn Tanner. Tanner writes extensively about cultural influences on theology. She stands firm in her thoughts that theology is a human construct. She goes further to say that the debates about theology between different theologians (see above with Brunner and Barth) are less about the truth of the interpretation of scriptures and more about competing cultural understandings. Because there is no one culture throughout the world, there is no one understanding of theology. As a result, a key theological task is to constantly reflect on what theologians are producing in order to analyze its veracity (in as much as possible). Tanner says we have far too often associated disagreements within Christianity as fights. Fights that lead to someone being right and someone being wrong. For reference to this type of behavior, we can once again visit Brunner and Barth. Barth's response to Brunner's theological musings is simply, NO! It does come across as petulant, but it also is a reflection of what can occur when theology is treated as either right or wrong. Tanner says we should be more akin to a learning community where we share ideas, disagreements, and agreements alike. It is through this task we inch closer to "seeing in part."

With this idea about the constructed nature of theology in place, I wanted to employ other theologians to help me come up with criteria by which we could start a learning community about good and bad theology. Peter Vardy and Duncan Ferguson deeply influenced the criteria with their respective texts, *Good and Bad Religion*[9] and *Exploring the Spirituality of the World Religions.*[10] Vardy is speaking broadly about the religions of the world when he discusses characteristics that are considered good and bad. At the center of Vardy's argument is that bad religion can consistently be traced to people who believe their religious conclusions are the only way

[8] 1 Corinthians 13:12, New Revised Standard Updated Version, Bible Gateway https://www.biblegateway.com/passage/?search=1+Corinthians+13%3A12&version=NRSVUE [accessed 4/6/24].

[9] Peter Vardy, *Good and Bad Religion* (London: SCM Press, 2010).

[10] Duncan Ferguson, *Exploring the Spirituality of the World Religions* (London: Continuum, 2010).

to believe. These folks are not willing to discuss their religion or their theology with others who disagree, but they hold steadfast to their understandings of the divine (and everything else). There is, of course, nothing wrong with believing one is correct about something as important as religion, but his problem comes when someone is so very convinced they are correct that they begin acting in ways that are damaging to others around them. Vardy also focuses on areas of justice and freedom. Religion, according to him, should empower humans to acts of justice and to encourage freedom and liberation. If one's religion is doing the opposite, then it is in the bad religion category for Vardy.

Ferguson talks specifically about spirituality in his text, and he has two categories of "life giving and life denying"[11] spirituality. In Ferguson's text, there are five aspects of spirituality that make it fall into either group. In life giving spirituality, you are empowered to live a good life. You are understanding and have compassion for your fellow human. Your goal is to make the world a better place than when you arrived. You are open to other people's thoughts and opinions on spirituality. Life giving spirituality is also there to support you in tough times. It sustains you and helps you navigate these inevitable parts of life. Life denying spirituality is the opposite of these things, in many ways. Your spirituality is closed off from the rest of the world. Not only are you closed off, but you are also judgmental to those who believe differently than yourself. There is no self-reflection about your beliefs (because they are right). There is enthusiasm in this type of spirituality, but it is enthusiasm for others to believe as you do (because you are right). Needless to say, these types of spirituality can be used by political parties or by religious leaders to convince people to join their causes. There is a definite "if you aren't with us, you are against us" about this type of spirituality.

With all of this preliminary heavy lifting done, I used ideas from my friends in order to create the criteria of good and bad theology. The criteria are as follows:

Good Theology

1. Your theology must relate to human flourishing. This inevitably will be defined in different ways, but people should feel as though their theology sustains, guides, and promotes them in a given context.

[11] Ferguson, *Exploring the Spirituality of the World Religions*, 10.

2. There must be space in your theology to self-reflect both at a personal level and at a community level.
3. Your theology should be open to hearing about the thoughts and beliefs of others even if they are different from your own thoughts and beliefs.
4. Alongside the openness to others, there should be freedom when it comes to an individual choosing their own theology.
5. There should be an openness to pursue justice in your theology. While this will look different depending on your context, there should exist in your theology a desire to liberate those who are oppressed.
6. Alongside the pursuit of justice, there should also be a desire for equality, both within one's tradition and outside in the secular world.

Bad Theology

1. Your theology is used to limit people's flourishing. This will inevitably be defined in different ways, but those oppressed under bad theology may feel they are not properly guided, sustained, or promoted in their given context.
2. There is little or no self-reflection in your theology. Instead, there is judgment on those who do not share the same theology.
3. There is no desire within your theology to interact with those who are outside your own community. In fact, there is an us versus them mentality when it comes to those who don't believe as you do.
4. Your theology is isolated from the rest of the world or from others who have a different theology from yours. Those within your community have little or no choice in their theology.
5. There is no desire for justice in the wider world in your theology, unless that justice fits within the already existing belief systems of your community.
6. There is no desire for equality in the wider world, unless that equality fits within already existing belief systems of your community.[12]

Because the criteria were created by me, with help from my theological friends, in a given time and a given place, they will no doubt evolve and change in the future. I want to hold my own theological conclusions to

[12] Robinson, *Bad Theology*, 65–66.

the same criteria that I adhere to for the sake of the overall project. Accordingly, I am not claiming that these criteria are true or right, but I do think that my conclusions could help in furthering conversations about how we understand theology.

A fun anecdote for any of my theology friends out there. My friend and fellow podcast theologian Kristy Whaley (Theology on the Rocks) heard some of my thoughts about this bad theology summary and shouted with glee, "Oh you're a Barthian!" I will not claim that, as unlike more legitimate systematic theologians, I have not read all the extensive writings of the man. But Barth is important to the overall conversation of theology in general, and as Kristy explained his thoughts on the importance of Jesus as our revelation of God in the world, and how the rest is our interpretations of these events throughout human history, I can see the connection. As Christians, we can believe in certain fundamentals as just that, but as those fundamentals extend into a wider conversation about the nature of God and the world, the waters get muddier. "But what are the fundamentals, Dr. Robinson?!" I will cheekily say, that firmly depends on who you are, I suppose.

A note about the system I have created. I was taught by many a great practical theologian about the importance of self-reflection. I am also a woman theologian, so I have inevitable moments of intense self-criticism. That being said, I'm aware that I have criteria about avoiding an us versus them mentality as well as limiting our practices of judging people, but it would seem that I have created a system of just that. I must argue that judging and even condemnation are inevitable in certain circumstances, especially in examples of things like slavery and genocide. That being said, up until this book I have only looked at historical examples that are widely viewed as evil in nature. It could be said that this is easy picking for a topic like this, and that would be absolutely correct. This was also a purposeful choice in terms of my previously mentioned examples. Calling the system of apartheid bad theology is not going to surprise anyone, nor will it amaze or dazzle theological students. That is because we have accepted that there are certain aspects of history that, widely speaking, are not justifiable by the human race. As I was first introducing the topic of bad theology, I was dipping my toe into the theological ocean by using examples that I had studied previously and that I had deemed as being bad theology (before the phrase even came into my head).

With the experiment out of the way and the book published and catching dust on the shelf, I decided to be a bit bolder in my approach. I wanted to stretch the muscles of my criterion to see how far we could go. This book is tackling topics that are still happening all around us right now or happened in the very immediate past. A phrase I always use when talking about bad theology is "one person's bad theology is another person's good theology." I stand by this as true. No one, not even the early Puritans who were murdering native peoples would have looked in the mirror and said, "You know what, this is some bad theology." That being said, the examples in the first book were so far away that we as a society could see that the theologically justified actions of some in history were bad theology. This project will be interesting in the sense that I will be talking about people who are still alive and who are still ministering in the here and now. These folks can, as the kids say, clap back at my assessment. Though based on the us versus them of most of them, I doubt they will ever read this book. In the meantime, you and I can talk about it. We can discuss and even debate, and instead of shouting NO! at one another, we can form a dialogical community that learns and grows together. That is the hope anyway. So, with criteria in place, we move towards the topic at hand. Pandemics have always been, and COVID-19 was certainly not the first, so I want to take you on a journey of some of the major pandemics throughout history before we dive into the current one. I would like the reader to begin the exercise of looking at the theological responses to pandemics in light of the bad theology criteria. This will get us prepped and ready for when we reach the current day and dig into the bad theology that ran/runs rampant in a COVID/post-COVID world.

CHAPTER 4

Theology and Pandemics: A History

> He tried to recall what he had read about the disease. Figures floated across his memory, and he recalled that some thirty or so great plagues known to history had accounted for nearly a hundred million deaths. But what are a hundred million deaths? When one has served in a war one hardly knows what a dead man is, after a while. And since a dead man has no substance unless one has actually seen him dead, a hundred million corpses broadcast through history are no more than a puff of smoke in the imagination.[1]

Lyman Stone writes in her article on March 13, 2020, that Christianity has been dealing with epidemics for 2000 years.[2] While some might debate that date, what we do know is that as long as Christianity has existed (formally and informally), there have been plagues and pandemics in the world. Accordingly, for as long as there have been pandemics and plagues, Christians have wrestled with how to respond theologically to something that appears so inherently counter-creation. The results have evolved through human history, but it is interesting in the case of this text to see that they by no means are uniform. This is important for a multitude of reasons, but for Bad Theology purposes, it is important because it

[1] Camus, *The Plague*, 38.

[2] Lyman Stone, "Christianity has been Handling Epidemics for 2000 years," Foreign Policy, https://foreignpolicy.com/2020/03/13/christianity-epidemics-2000-years-should-i-still-go-to-church-coronavirus/ [accessed 2/15/24].

L. Robinson, *Bad Theology in a Time of COVID*,
https://doi.org/10.1007/978-3-031-75294-0_4

highlights that theological understandings of pandemics and plagues have changed as society has changed. The idea that there has been one, unified, God-given response to pandemics and plagues in the world is a myth. Further giving evidence to the idea that theology is a human, social construct, we see that theology shifted in terms of its response to diseases in the world. Also, there is a clear, if not evolving, trajectory of theological responses that led us to 2020 and the COVID-19 virus. I am a theologian, but I do firmly believe that history teaches us a great deal about ourselves in the present. This can be culturally, geographically, or ethnically, but it can also be theologically. So, in terms of Christian history, I am starting at the beginning.

The Early Church

N.T. Wright, in his book *God and the Pandemic*,[3] describes the response to disasters and their consequent devastation in the ancient, European world. In ancient Greco-Roman times, things like disease, earthquakes, fires, death, and so on were all associated with angry gods. If disasters happen upon a person, it is most inevitably because they did something to anger someone or some deity. That being said, the philosophers of this world felt that simply blaming folks "up there" was not a very critical way to view the world and what happened in the world. These ancient philosophers created schools of thought about what happened to humans while they were in the earthly realm. According to Wright: "First the Stoics. Everything is programmed to turn out the way it does. You can't change it; just learn to fit in. Alternatively, the Epicureans Everything is random. You can't do anything. Make yourself as comfortable as you can. Then the Platonists. The present life is just a shadow of reality. Bad things happen here but we are destined for a different world."[4] Keep these ancient thoughts in mind because they have not left the contemporary way of thinking about COVID-19. Back to the timeline, though.

In the early days of formalizing Christianity, after Jesus' death and with multitudes of texts about his life floating around, you had councils full of learned men who set themselves the task of defining the tradition. What I have learned through many years of teaching world religions is that the major world religions all had a time period of what I call "assembling."

[3] Tom Wright, *God and the Pandemic* (London: SPCK, 2020).

[4] Wright, *God and the Pandemic*, 2.

This time period is when the leader of the new religion is out of the picture and what remains are accounts of their life and teachings. It is during the assembling time that those who adhere to the new religion come together and decide what is a legit text or teaching and also what the main tenets of the religion will be. It can sound very clinical in practice, and I can bet it was so in real life. Christianity was no different. Three hundred years or so after Jesus' death, there was a feeling that Christianity needed to be reeled in, for lack of a better phrase. There needed to be an account of the "actual" texts of the tradition and the "actual" theology that believers should adhere to in order to be considered orthodox. The Councils of Nicea (325 A.D.), Constantinople (381 A.D.), and Chalcedon (451 A.D.) were just the place to solidify the who, what, where, and when of Christianity. The biblical canon was sealed, the divinity of Jesus was confirmed, theological concepts like the Trinity were created, and salvation was clarified and systematized.

During this time period, there were parallel scientific movements that were also being confirmed as "canon," if you will. The history of medicine is basically the history of humanity. Much like religion, as long as we have records of humans practicing some form of religion, you also have humans attempting to use the surrounding world for helping and healing. Starting with Hippocrates, and furthered by work by Galen, the medical sciences progressed significantly during the time period of the early Christian church. Hippocrates speculated that to maintain health in a human, there must be a balance of four humors that are a part of the human body: "the 4 most common humors: blood, phlegm, yellow bile, and black … Each of the humors corresponded with one of the 4 elements, air corresponded to blood, water to phlegm, earth to black bile, and fire to yellow bile."[5] In Hippocrates' theory, humans became sick when their humors were out of balance. Treatments for sickness leaned into treatments that would lead the humors back into a balanced state. There were many other theories circulating at the time about what caused disease and sickness, but the most important development in this time period was around the idea that external (or divine) forces were not necessarily at play in causing someone to feel unwell. To these modern scientists, the answer to ailments was within the body itself. Treatment, therefore, was also focused on the body, primarily.

[5] Paul Dansereau, Austin Mardon, Catherine Mardon, *Pandemic Theology* (Edmonton: Golden Meteorite Press, 2020), 12.

In order to see how far of a development this was in terms of how people saw disease and sickness, one needs to look only to the Greek poet Homer. Homer predates Hippocrates by several centuries. His views within his two masterpieces, the *Illiad* and the *Odyssey*, offer a window into the views of medicine in the Greco-Roman world during this time. The Greeks of Homer's time would have seen sickness and the divine as being inherently linked. In Homer's works, there are illnesses that occur from the physical world (like injury from beasts or plants etc.), but there are also distinct disasters that occur as a result of the gods being angered. At the beginning of the *Illiad*, Apollo sends down a plague on humanity. This is a common origin for negative occurrences that are so catastrophic in scope that there is no physical explanation for them. "When the ancient Greeks did conclude that a disease or a disaster was from the Gods, their explanation for it often echoed what many people throughout history thought: that people were being punished for angering a divinity."[6]

During the time of the early church, when so many theological ideas were being written into the canon, you also get the development of a new, non-theological way of viewing science. Despite the differences in scientific theories at the time, there were some commonalities that challenged the authority of the church. "Hippocratic physicians shared in common the view of and approach to medicine as a natural, physical phenomenon independent of divinity, and able to be explained and treated through logic and understanding."[7] The change in views during this time period meant that the authority of the church as a means of healing and curing illnesses shifted significantly from the pews to the hospital ward. For many, this was a new and challenging idea, but for others, it was a welcome challenge to the exclusivity that the church had long held on those seeking wellness. Prior to this time period, the church was seen as the end-all place to get your ailments treated and fixed. God was the one who was the creator as well as the healer and restorer. The church, as a result, was the conduit of this healing. The new developments in the scientific method of this era shifted this primacy of the church to that of the medical world. It did not take away the church as an aspect of healing, but the scientific community saw it as just one aspect of the holistic understanding of a human.

[6] Dansereau et al., *Pandemic Theology*, 10.
[7] Dansereau et al., *Pandemic Theology*, 14.

> [The author of the Hippocratic text *The Sacred Disease*] has no issues with the practices of praying and sacrificing to the Gods, or with those individuals who serve or choose to seek healing at temples–the author instead attacks 'those who claim to be able to drive out demons and compel the Gods to do their will by means of chants and charm,' as *where in temples the decision of healing is ultimately left to the will of the Gods themselves, these individuals claim a personal relationship with the divine as well as power to use this relationship to heal upon their command.*[8]

As mentioned previously, the physician Galen took over the methods of Hippocrates and made them into his own image in the first century. Galen furthered ideas around the area of surgery and various other areas of internal medicine. At one point, he was so well known in the region that he was called upon to work on the Gladiators when they were injured in battle. Arguably, his most influential contribution to this time period was that of his understanding of the human anatomy. Understanding of the internal body had been somewhat frowned upon in the Greco-Roman world, but Galen knew that knowledge of the makeup of the body was key to treating illness. Interestingly enough, despite Galen's advances in scientific methods, he still maintained a dualistic approach to healing. He believed there was "a benevolent Creator who put herbs and medicine in the world so that humanity could use them to relieve suffering-a notion easily compatible with belief in the Christian God."[9] Many priests, who were known to be learned individuals, also operated as medical doctors during this time. In fact, Galen helped to explain how it was not a heresy for priests to work in the medicinal world. God put the elements in the world to help people to be healed, and as a result, God was healing people through God's followers on earth who were able to wield such blessings in their favor.

So, while all of this development was happening in science, we return now to the early church. One might think that the de-centralization of the church as the ultimate healer in the Roman Empire would have caused a major decline in interest, but instead what we see is the church adopting a new role in sickness and disease. Prior to the legalization of Christianity in the Roman Empire in 313 AD, the Christian community was operating undercover, largely. During this time of hiding, Christians began building "Diaconia" structures that served the sick and dying. Many scholars see

[8] Dansereau et al., *Pandemic Theology*, 16. Emphasis author's.

[9] Dansereau et al., *Pandemic Theology*, 22.

these buildings as early hospitals. With the legalization of Christianity, these buildings multiplied and diversified. By 369 AD, St Basil of Caesarea had responded to the call by those who were increasingly ill and needing care through the founding of a building with 300 beds for the sick and dying. This is oftentimes considered the first official hospital in the Roman Empire. What was the need for such a large institution to care for the sick and dying? It will be familiar to many a reader. It is to the Black Death that we turn our attention next.

Black Death

When one thinks of pandemics, outside of our current situation, the mind will often go directly to the Black Death. The height of the Black Death was between 1347 and 1351 and it was responsible for the deaths of somewhere in the realm of one-fourth to half of Europe's entire population at the time. Numbers are hard to imagine in times like this, and indeed, they are sometimes just as hard to count accurately. Many a conspiracy theorists throughout history would say this is because of contrived danger in the face of pandemics, but a more historical way to view this issue in counting is that it is just plain difficult. People in different areas of the world and in different parts of society handle sickness and death in a variety of ways. This variety means that unless they are going through official measures (usually medical/governmental), there might not be a register of their death at all. Add to that some communities who are suspicious of authorities or some with just no access to official means of registering death, and one begins to see the inherent difficulties in accounting for widespread death. In the Black Death, the range is huge, 20 to 100 million deaths estimated from various sources. If we take a more conservative stance of around 25 million for instance, it still means that in those years mentioned as the height of the pandemic, there were 14,000 people dying per day in Europe. Per day. From an overall population level, the Black Death and the famines that followed reduced the population of Europe from 440 million to 350 million (estimates).[10]

I won't dive into the science intensely, but it is worth noting what caused such a disastrous situation in Europe. The Black Death was an infectious disease caused by a bacterium called Y. Pestis. Historically, science has defined "plague" as being a sickness caused by this specific

[10] Dansereau et al., *Pandemic Theology*, 33.

bacterium. How a human catches this bacterium is how one knows what kind of plague they have. So, for instance, bubonic plague is from insects that spread the sickness from one infected animal to the next via bites. Pneumonic plague is spread by inhaling the bacteria into your lungs. This is spread from person to person. The final form of plague is called septicemic plague, which is an infection of the blood. This is the rarest form of plague. It is certainly possible to see multiple forms of the plague in one person. By the end of the story, we see this in Camus' *The Plague*.

One other thing to note about the Black Death in Europe is that the population was not prepared to fight this outbreak. It was not the first plague to hit Europe, there were others that were recorded. The one of significance that was nearest in time to the Black Death was called the Plague of Justinian (541–549 AD). There are differing accounts of how significant this plague was in Europe (see above about reporting deaths and numbers), but what we do know is that it was a noteworthy and extremely deadly plague. Many would argue it matched the Black Death in its death tolls. The Plague of Justinian was especially catastrophic in Constantinople. During this time, the advisor to Emperor Justinian I, Procopius, writes the following:

> Dear but for this calamity it is quite impossible either to express in words or to conceive in thought any explanation, except indeed to refer it to God. For it did not come in a part of the world nor upon certain men, nor did it confine itself to any season of the year, so that from such circumstances it might be possible to find subtle explanations of a cause, but it embraced the entire world, and blighted the lives of all men, though differing from one another in the most marked degree, respecting neither sex nor age.[11]

So, while many historians of that time would say the Black Death was the second plague of its kind in Europe, the facts remain that the population was not prepared for the second any more than it was for the first. There has been speculation about why this might have been the case. Europe was no stranger to disasters, and alongside plagues, there were also famines and wars (most notably the 100 Years War between France and England that ravaged the land). And yet, they were still no more prepared for death, disease, and war than if none had ever existed prior. Your author does not feel that is the fault of Europe, nor any country that goes through

[11] Dansereau et al., *Pandemic Theology*, 33.

such things. It is my opinion that humans can only handle a certain amount of things at a time being thrown at them. Oftentimes, we are attempting to not sink, despite looking very much like we are casually floating. As a result, it is a very optimistic view to think that Europe could have been overly prepared for the Black Death, as parts of Europe were battling each other during the height of the outbreak. Now, what leaders do once these disasters strike, your author is less kind about, but we will see more to that later.

By most accounts, the Black Death originated in Asia. The European brand of plague was found in fleas in central Asia living among local rat populations. Also, much like a storm system, you can see the slow but unsettling movement of the plague across countries. In China, India, and other parts of Asia, approximately 25 million people died. That being said, what was once a disease whispered about as happening "over there" had eventually become a very real "here" problem for Europeans in 1347. Ships sailing from eastern Europe to Constantinople carried the disease on board. By the end of 1347, the plague was seen throughout France and Italy. As the year 1350 rolled around, Europe was properly in the grip of the plague.

Scientists and theologians alike were interested in explaining the effective devastation that was happening around them. For most members of European society, this horror could not just be a matter of chance. While the link to fleas in far-off lands would come much later, there were theories that floated around at the time. One of the more popular understandings of how the plague began was that there was some issue with the air that caused people's humors (see Hippocrates) to be out of balance and eventually led them to fall ill. The other side of there being bad air, naturally, is there must be good air. The people of this time used to adorn themselves with flowers and sweet-smelling things in order to ward off the bad air and surround themselves with good air. A less earthly theory circulating at this time was that the plague occurred because the planets were out of line. In many ways, that theory combined some science and some extra-terrestrial elements to the disease. Those who were in religious communities began to point fingers at other religious communities for the plague, which is both surprising and not surprising in many ways. Christians, most famously, blamed the Jewish populations for the outbreaks. This caused a great deal of violence and anti-Semitic rhetoric to pervade Europe and lead to further anti-Semitic actions that would weave themselves throughout the history of Europe (to this day).

In summary, Europeans had theories of what was going on, but none of them were even close to right. As a result, the plague swept through the continent and destroyed all in its path. All the while, the population was pointing fingers at dirty air, other religious groups, and the planets. Needless to say, the disease thrived in this scenario. When the plague eventually ran its course, there were new issues to deal with. By 1351, the plague had slowed down, but this was not the end of the story. If we learned anything from COVID-19, it was that the conclusion of the outbreak is not the end of the story by a long shot. So it was in Europe, with populations being so decreased there were widespread worker shortages. Even if the workers were not ill or dead at this stage, they were still living in fear of the past five years. As a result, workers (especially in rural areas) became a hot commodity, and those in the workforce swiftly found this out. Though there were attempts by wealthy landowners to keep this movement down, the workers found themselves in positions of power that they had never experienced before.

The plagues of Europe would continue, but never to the degree of the Black Death. Scientifically and theologically, there was a lot of reflection about the plague in its aftermath.

> Beyond the Black Death the plague became less of an apocalyptic act of God and more of a source of general anxiety and fear. It was during one of these outbreaks in 1377 that the term 'quarantine' was created. In Ragusa (modern day Dubrovnik, Croatia), the city's council established a law requiring those visiting the city to remain in a *trentino*, a thirty-day period of isolation, which was eventually lengthened to a forty-day *quarantino*.[12]

During the seventeenth and eighteenth centuries, you begin to get the illustration of the masked and heavily clothed plague doctor. While this image is often used in relation to horror imagery-some historians argue if it was a real-life image or a theater image. There is an idea that at the very least doctors were becoming incredibly superstitious about what actually caused the plague, but still with an emphasis on good air. As a result of some of these doctor's often experimental and usually superstitious methods, the plague did slowly lose some of its veracity. Also, general improvements in Europe in sanitation and living situations meant that a second Black Death never occurred.

[12] Dansereau et al., *Pandemic Theology*, 41.

Plagues did not disappear completely, however. It seemed to always be hiding just below the surface waiting for humans to grow complacent in some way. In the 1800s and 1900s, there were several more outbreaks of the plague, but by this time there were scientific developments about where the plague came from and how to treat it, at least in Europe. By 1855, scientists Kitasto Shibasaburo and Alexandre Yerstin had both discovered the bacterium that was the origin of the plague. In 1854, Paul Louis Simon published a paper about how the plague spread from rats to fleas to humans. During this time period, there were only 457 deaths in Europe from the plague. In contrast, in 1896, a plague swept India and killed almost 12 million people. Moving forward in history, it became increasingly clear that the plague was most damaging to people who didn't have the developments in the causes of the spread of the plague, most notably sanitation, clean living standards, and governmental bodies that would require limits on interactions amongst people (like quarantines).[13]

I have spoken a great deal about the history of the Black Death, including scientific developments. We turn now to the religious implications of the Black Death on Europe, specifically. We discussed earlier that by the 1300s, Christianity had already lost a great deal of influence on the overall population of Europe. This is not to say there was not a desire for the church to guide society, but there was not a reliance on the church to do this. This singular reliance had split and shifted to the study of science, societal advancement, astronomy, and medicine (to name a few). So, by the time of the Black Plague, the church was important, but it was not vital to the continuation of society in Europe at this time.

When the plague struck, the Catholic church was not immune to its devastation. If anything, its clergy were hit worse because of people's desire to have priests present in their final moments of living. It just so happened that during the plague, their final moments of living meant that they were contagious with an illness that people could not explain. McLaurine Zentner discusses this in their work: *The Black Death and Its Impact on the Church and Popular Religion*. Zentner details the numbers that were collected for clergy deaths during this period. "During the height of the plague in 1349, roughly 45 percent of the priests in 10 dioceses throughout England died ... one of highest rates of mortality recorded among priests during the Black Death was in the diocese of

[13] Dansereau et al., *Pandemic Theology*, 41–42.

Barcelona, where it reached 60 percent between 1348 and 1349."[14] This gives two windows into the deaths of clergy (and doctors) in Europe during this time who were expected to be at the front line of the crisis. The large gap that was left by these deaths meant that there was a recruitment campaign for the ordination of priests. Inevitably, with such extreme demand and such low supply, quality of priests slipped significantly. Even though many people trusted science and advancement, when they were confronted with the reality of death, they wanted to get their eternal matters in order. As a result, priests performing last rites were in high demand. The low quality of priests in some of these scenarios certainly did not endear the local population to that of the Catholic church, but the British phrase, "needs must" seemed to prevail on both sides of the altar. A theological response from within the church to the plague is a common conclusion in such times. The plague was a result of the sinful behavior of humanity. The deaths and disease were a direct result of God's wrath upon Europe. Conveniently, this sin can be attributed to the people's move away from the church as a center of society in Europe at this time. It is a self-serving theology for the church, and a rather impractical way to explain away diseases, but so it was.

Moving to the practical theology of it all, it is important to give a bit of background on how it was to die in Europe during this time.

> The *ars moriendi*, or art of dying, was an important tradition for European Christians that helped them prepare for the journey after death. Confessions and the giving of last rites were an important part of this tradition … These rituals and sacramental services were important because they allowed the Church to help calm the fear of death among European Christians, but priests struggled to perform them effectively in the wake of the plague.[15]

Interestingly, though theology is often argued as an unchanging and objective narrative, it shifted significantly in light of the plague. It gave theology the appearance of being a social construct that is adaptable to time and place, an argument long held by your author. Practically

[14] McLaurine Zentner, *The Black Death and Its Impact on the Church and Popular Religion*, Honor's Thesis, University of Mississippi (2015), 5 https://egrove.olemiss.edu/cgi/viewcontent.cgi?article=1682&context=hon_thesis [accessed 3/7/24].

[15] Zentner, *The Black Death and Its Impact on the Church and Popular Religion*, Honor's Thesis, University of Mississippi (2015), 9 https://egrove.olemiss.edu/cgi/viewcontent.cgi?article=1682&context=hon_thesis [accessed 3/7/24].

speaking, with priests being at a minimum and people still desiring last rites, the theological underpinning of last rites shifted. Bishop Shrewsbury of Bath and Wells, in 1349, declared that Christians were able to die without the sacrament of penance and still reach heaven. Confession was still important, however, and the bishop stated that people could confess to a layperson. This confession would be recognized, presumably by the church, but also by heavenly bodies. A delightful ending to this decree is that Christians could confess to any lay person, really. Even a woman if a man was not around to do so.[16]

Another religious reaction during the plague was that of a group known as the Flagellants. The act of whipping oneself was not new in Christian history and its origins are dated as far back as the fifth century. That being said, it was seen as an extreme practice of penance by those who participated. Radical, but not in the way you might want to be known as radical. Why did this movement become popular in the midst of the Black Death? The answer lies in the theological understanding of why the plague had happened. According to the Flagellants, "believing the plague to be a result of sin, the extreme penance undertaken was believed to elicit mercy and forgiveness from God."[17] The Flagellants would organize themselves and parade through the streets of towns whipping themselves and proclaiming their repentance in light of the current plague. The movement was met with relative support from the people, who I would imagine, were willing to try just about anything to see if it would stop the illness. Alongside their public displays, they would also preach and prophesy. They believed that the plague was a key event and marked the immanent return of Jesus to earth. In both preaching and prophesy, they undermined the Catholic church and its teachings. The pope at the time, Clement VI, was less than impressed with this display of penance, which he saw as being more about parading oneself in public and superstition than actual belief in God. In the decrees from the Catholic church against these radicals, there is an underlying feeling of a fearful church that was rapidly losing influence on its congregants in the midst of disaster. The flagellants went so far as to say they could forgive sins, and in many ways, this was the last straw for the larger church. The church has never been

[16] Zentner, *The Black Death and Its Impact on the Church and Popular Religion,* Honor's Thesis, University of Mississippi (2015), 10 https://egrove.olemiss.edu/cgi/viewcontent.cgi?article=1682&context=hon_thesis [Accessed 3/7/24].

[17] Dansereau et al., *Pandemic Theology*, 49.

good at sharing power, and this was a prime example of someone challenging it.[18]

A final religious reaction to the plague was discrimination and hate. Anti-Jewish sentiment prevailed throughout the plague (and prior and after) in Europe. This came to a particular head in Southern France during the time of the Black Death whereby Jews were blamed for the illness that pervaded the area. Specifically, according to stories of the time, the true cause of the plague was Jewish people poisoning the wells. This is a combination of extreme scapegoating and a view of the Jews as being mystical in some way. This was not a new fight for Jews in Europe. They had a distinct culture, lived in community, had a distinct way of dressing, were successful in areas of finance, and ultimately (in the eyes of some Christians), they had rejected the message of Jesus when it was presented. All of these aspects, either real or imagined, created an anti-Semitic view of the Jews that meant when something bad happened, they were the culprit.[19] The Black Death was no different. Pope Clement, again, tried to quell the violence that was erupting against the Jews throughout Europe, but to no avail. "The Pope represented the entire institution of the Church, and it is noteworthy that his public word did nothing to calm the hysteria that had taken control of Europe. Individuals lost faith in the ability of the clergy to guide them through the disaster of the plague, and most Christians refused to heed their demands for the protection of the Jews."[20] By the last years of the plague, Jews were being killed in many countries in Europe, and at a rapid rate, mostly through burning, and in some cases, public drowning and other forms of murder. Despite the Pope's pleas, the intensity of the local population's feelings against the Jewish population could not be stopped. Even some clergy got in on the anti-Semitism, encouraging the rumors and stories about Jews in their local congregations. It is a significant tragedy in the history of the plague, and it is one of terrible foreshadowing for the years to come. The European population was searching for the meaning behind the plague, the alternative being that there is no meaning, and they are living in a world where things just

[18] Zentner, *The Black Death and Its Impact on the Church and Popular Religion,* Honor's Thesis, University of Mississippi (2015), 34–37 https://egrove.olemiss.edu/cgi/viewcontent.cgi?article=1682&context=hon_thesis [Accessed 3/7/24].

[19] Dansereau et al., *Pandemic Theology*, 50.

[20] Zentner, *The Black Death and Its Impact on the Church and Popular Religion,* Honor's Thesis, University of Mississippi (2015), 43–44 https://egrove.olemiss.edu/cgi/viewcontent.cgi?article=1682&context=hon_thesis [Accessed 3/7/24].

happen. For many, this was an unacceptable reality. This in no way excuses the violence and absolute vile hatred towards the Jews. It, in fact, highlights what humanity becomes when they are left without any societal structures that once framed their life. Inhuman, it would appear.

The Spanish Flu

We move now to another major pandemic that wrecked the world with its veracity, the Spanish Flu. Unlike the plague, there is actually little known about the origins of this virus. This, mixed with its beginnings in World War I, meant that the Spanish Flu was chaotic from the beginning. The term "flu" comes from the Italian word for "influenced," as there was a belief at this time that the stars had a direct correlation to the issues that existed on earth.[21] Since the sixteenth century, we have seen pandemics of the influenza virus throughout history, periodically popping up in various geographical locations. At the time of the Spanish Flu, however, there was a limited understanding of what caused the virus and its spread. Now, we are aware there are Type A and B flu viruses, Type A being the virus strand that is responsible for pandemics. Another important aspect of the flu virus is that when the body fights a virus, it can produce mutations of the original virus or viruses. This is a process called reassortant. This was an important cause of death in the Spanish Flu epidemic, where there were up to 200 different strands of the virus at a given time. So, even when our bodies fight a strand of a virus, it can change, and if we catch it again, it can be as though we never had it to begin with. Of course, in the pandemic of 1918, this information was not known. It would be another decade and a half before the flu virus was identified and studied thoroughly. What is known, looking back, is that there was a lack of information about the virus, but there was also a world war that was raging in Europe that caused less than sanitary or healthful conditions for people in general. This created a perfect storm for the Spanish Flu pandemic.[22]

As mentioned previously, there is no real indication of the origin of the Spanish Flu. There are two theories that are tossed around in regard to the recorded beginnings of the outbreak. In Kansas (USA), a mess cook came down with the virus while on a military base in 1918. Albert Gitchell, the cook, was known as patient zero, although all we really know is that he was

[21] Dansereau et al., *Pandemic Theology*, 54.
[22] Dansereau et al., *Pandemic Theology*, 55-56.

the first recorded case of this pandemic. Another theory about the origins of the virus was that it began in a northern province of China. In 1917, Dr. Wu Lein-teh, a doctor who had battled a previous plague in China, was deeply concerned to hear of a sickness dubbed "The Winter Sickness" that was afflicting the local population. People were not dying at nearly the rate of the previous plague outbreak, however, and the government was quick to discredit the doctor's concerns.

A final collection of origins of the Spanish Flu are directly related to the war itself. Various military bases in France that housed both British and Chinese fighters began to experience sicknesses that were akin to the flu. This created a great deal of finger-pointing as to who was bringing the virus and from where. The answers to this may never be known, but what is known is the war created a mass movement of people from different parts of the world to other parts. This is a prime situation for any virus that hopes to spread throughout the world, and so it did. By the end of the war, there were theories that the virus began in the USA, Britain, China, France, and even Russia. With the movement of people and the distraction of war, it will most likely never be known where it began. And to some degree, it does not matter in the end. The pandemic happened, and it was the worst the world had seen, no matter where it began.[23]

The accounts of those who died from the Spanish Flu, much like the plague, differ depending on who you ask. As explained previously, this is common during the chaos of a widespread illness, not to mention mixing in a world war. Some people say, at the least, it was 25 million, and the numbers rise to 50 million with others. Still others say the number is closer to 100 million. The estimated deaths can be frustrating for some modern readers who want exact numbers, but even in our contemporary world, the numbers we have following pandemics are still estimates, despite our recording devices becoming more advanced for such things.

The Spanish Flu was unusual in a sense because it occurred over the course of three distinct time periods. It was not a continuous pandemic. The first of these periods began in March 1918. The second period began in the summer of that year and lasted until December. Finally, the last time period began in January. In the midst of these time periods, you have troops moving across different locations, and you even have the end of the war itself. The name, the Spanish Flu, was not nearly as helpful in its description as it might appear. Spain did not have any real claims to the

[23] Dansereau et al., *Pandemic Theology*, 57–58.

start of the pandemic or even the most cases throughout the different time periods. What it did have was neutrality during World War I, and that meant it was freer to report on news that was not necessarily positive in nature (a practice that was frowned upon by warring nations during this time period). Spain was thus able to report about the flu, its outbreaks, and the devastation it was causing globally. Hence, the rest of the world began to dub the virus the Spanish Flu, and the name stuck.[24]

The virus spread across the world, and as mentioned previously, the movement of soldiers in light of World War I did not help the situation. In the first period of the flu, we see something similar to a lot of pandemics. The virus hit vulnerable groups the hardest, with the young and the elderly being especially vulnerable. The second time period, however, was strange in its delivery. Those who were hardest hit were the healthiest, those between the ages of 20 and 40. The defense that the healthiest bodies had against the virus was actually its own undoing, as people fell ill due to their own body's reaction against the virus, such as inflammation. Women were also affected at a much higher rate than in the previous time period of the virus. Amazingly, 1918 became the first year in recorded history where there were more deaths than births.

The flu itself spread much like the flu we know today. Droplets from breath or direct contact would spread the virus from person to person. In the initial period of the virus, the symptoms were very flu-like. People would get sore throats, headaches, body aches, and feel generally worn down. By the second wave, however, the symptoms had become more severe with skin discoloration as well as the loss of hair and teeth. The second and third waves also saw the flu causing further problems in the people it infected by way of pneumonia.[25]

Reactions to the Spanish Flu, globally, make for an interesting analysis, especially in light of the ongoing war at the time. While the Spanish Flu claimed more lives than World War I, it seemed that global powers were far more concerned about the war than anything else. For example, "In England, despite the efforts of a mathematician named Major Greenwood to warn officials of the impending second wave, all he received for his efforts were derision, as individuals such as the General Medical Council representative and Army Sanitary Committee representative Sir Arthur Newsholme dismissed his concerns, as he felt it was more important to

[24] Dansereau et al., *Pandemic Theology*, 58–59.
[25] Dansereau et al., *Pandemic Theology*, 60–61.

keep the country functioning and to prioritize the war effort."[26] The United States was not much better. In New York City, President Woodrow Wilson was allowed to lead a parade of 25,000 people through the city. That same week, NYC saw 2000 people die from Spanish Flu. In Philadelphia, the city officials basically denied the existence of the flu, and as a result, they were responsible for more deaths than the heavily populated NYC.[27]

One of the interesting after-effects of the Spanish Flu was in relation to mental health. There were global increases in depression, anxiety, and general sense of loss. This, combined with the consequences of the war, caused a general malaise in the global population. A further development was how little people were willing to actually speak about the Spanish Flu despite its devastating effect on the world.

> One of the strangest things about the legacy of the Spanish Flu is the lack of one. Theories as to why vary; some suggest that it was a forgotten in a conscious attempt to dull the pain caused; others suggest it was overshadowed by the war for one reason or another; and other still argue that, perhaps it wasn't any sort of intentional purge or silence at all, but was instead simply the natural reaction of a world that had already suffered more than it could bear.[28]

The theological responses to the Spanish Flu were far different than that of the Black Death. By the time the Spanish Flu hit, the world had moved to a different space in its relationship with science and religion. Post Enlightenment, there was a (albeit false) dichotomy between the world of science and religion. It was not that Euro-America had given up religion necessarily, but more that the church did not hold all the answers to all the questions of the world. In some ways, this decreased the influence of the church on pandemics in the day-to-day. In other ways, it increased thinking about the deeper theological questions about the role of God in the world, including the classic question of why bad things happen to good people.

One aspect of the theology of the Spanish Flu that was consistent with the Black Death was questions regarding God's part (or not) in the pandemic. The answers to these questions oftentimes depended greatly on

[26] Dansereau et al., *Pandemic Theology*, 62.
[27] Dansereau et al., *Pandemic Theology*, 62–63.
[28] Dansereau et al., *Pandemic Theology*, 65.

denominational affiliation. An example out of South Africa, the Presbyterians in the region were certain that God had a direct hand in the virus and its spread. Most non-Calvinists in the region were less convinced of this and cited that the virus came about because of social reasons. Poverty, and the lack of sanitation and provisions associated with finances, was the reason behind the virus and its spread, according to this community. If humans were being punished, it was not the direct hand of God because of sin, but because of humanity's lack of care for their neighbors. Catholics in the region referred directly to "nature"[29] as being the reason the Spanish Flu had taken over so affectively, but gave little further explanation. It was arguably tough theological and mental gymnastics. Even before Leonard Cohen, there were theological questions about an interventionist God and the level of intervention in this interventionist God. You can see that playing out in this debate about the Spanish Flu (and consequent pandemics). Did God cause this? Why? If so, can God stop it? Will God protect believers? If a believer dies what does this say about God if God caused this? What if God isn't involved at all? And so on.

In the midst of these abstract debates about God were the debates about the practicality of what the Spanish Flu meant for those who were churchgoers in regions that were hit especially hard. Returning to South Africa, we see debates beginning to arise about whether it was safe (or responsible) to attend churches. There were many local bans on gatherings that were inside, which would include religious services of any kind. The responses from the clergy were anything but neutral. Calvinists in the area were especially concerned that the ban limited communal activities in a time where they are most needed.

> Most Anglican ministers also expressed themselves in favour of continuing regular services, either because it was a time when people were looking to their religion in particular for help and comfort or because not to do so would imply that appealing to God communally was useless in such circumstances. Some clergymen tried to resolve their dilemma by shortening services or holding them out of doors, but many ignored the ban, pointing to the non-closure of gathering places like bars, shops, and markets.[30]

[29] Howard Phillips, "Why Did It Happen?: Religious Explanations of the 'Spanish' Flu Epidemic In South Africa," in *Historically Speaking* (September/October 2008), 35.

[30] Howard Phillips, "Why Did It Happen?: Religious Explanations of the 'Spanish' Flu Epidemic In South Africa," in *Historically Speaking* (September/October 2008), 35.

Local governments were slow to enforce the ban on gatherings at churches, though they were content enough to hold other gatherings to account. In a rather amusing theological move, a certain Congregationalist chaplain declared that if the church ban was not going to be enforced then bans on cinemas and theaters should also not be enforced. The logic of this argument was questioned by local clergy who could not believe that someone who had intimate knowledge of the importance of the church would make such a comparison between the physical and the spiritual, but the argument was now out in the world. What role does the government have in the regulation of religious services?

Elsewhere, in North America, the ban on public gatherings during the Spanish Flu was largely obeyed in Canada and the United States. If anything, the closing of churches in North America strengthened feelings of appreciation for the institution itself. People missed their weekly gatherings and there were public reflections about how the church itself was taken for granted until this time period when it was unavailable. Clergy published sermons in local newspapers and encouraged their congregations to host their own services, of sorts, in their homes. This included reading the sermons and having communal prayer as a household. One Presbyterian minister in Washington D.C., Rev. Francis Grimke, delivered a sermon reflecting on the closing of the churches after they had reopened. Grimke reiterated the necessity of all public gatherings to be closed in order to ensure the protection of the wider community, and he praised the commissioners who came to the conclusion to shut down certain places of community. He states:

> Another thing that has impressed me in connection with this epidemic, is the fact that conditions may arise in a community which justify the extraordinary exercise of powers that would not be tolerated under ordinary circumstances. This extraordinary exercise of power was resorted to by the Commissioners in closing up the theaters, schools, churches, in forbidding all gatherings of any considerable number of people indoors and outdoors, and in restricting the numbers who should be present even at funerals. The ground of the exercise of this extraordinary power was found in the imperative duty of the officials to safeguard, as far as possible, the health of the community by preventing the spread of the disease from which we suffer.[31]

[31] John Pellowe, "How the Church Responded to Previous Pandemics" Canadian Centre for Christian Charities, January 11, 2021 https://www.cccc.org/news_blogs/john/2021/01/11/how-the-church-responded-to-previous-pandemics/ [accessed 5/1/23].

Public disobedience against the ordinances related to the Spain Flu in North America was limited, but not zero. In 1919 San Francisco, there were 100 people who were charged for not wearing masks. There was even an organization called "The Anti-Mask League of San Francisco" that held a meeting with 2,000 people in attendance. The league was focused on the mask requirements throughout the city at the time. Another protest came from two Christian Scientist churches. One church claimed that "the police power of the state should not be used to prevent Christian worship in the churches."[32] What this highlights is that many arguments concerning the legality of closing religious institutions (and its relation to the freedom of religion section of the First Amendment) were debated in North America during the Spanish Flu. That being said, the overwhelming majority of churches and churchgoers adhered to the laws in place for the protection of the community.

HIV/AIDS

Another example of a global pandemic that bridges the gap from times that seem distant memory to where we are in 2024 is HIV/AIDS. The viral crisis that occurred predominately in the 1980s/90s. I bring up this example because it is here where we start to see the human population consumed not only by the disease, but by politics, religion, and fear mongering. A fear mongering that will be easily recognizable to those who have survived the pandemic that is COVID-19.

HIV represents the moniker given to the Human Immunodeficiency Virus. The virus attacks white blood cells in the body and renders humans less able to defend themselves against infections that might occur in their day-to-day life. The virus infects healthy white blood cells and copies itself in order to make more of the virus. Eventually, the virus takes over the body completely, and when a person's white blood cell count (specifically the CD4 T cells) falls below 200 per microliter of blood, they are diagnosed with AIDS (Acquired Immune Deficiency Syndrome). As a result,

[32] John Pellowe, "How the Church Responded to Previous Pandemics" Canadian Centre for Christian Charities, January 11, 2021 https://www.cccc.org/news_blogs/john/2021/01/11/how-the-church-responded-to-previous-pandemics/ [accessed 5/1/23].

AIDS patients typically die from infections that most people would be able to defend easily, but with the CD4 T cells so depleted, they simply cannot.[33]

The virus had existed prior to the 1980s, but it was during this time that attention was drawn to the increasing number of patients. In the beginning, it was seen as a disease that predominately affected gay men. This community was dying at a rapid rate from infections that healthy, young, men should be able to fight off. In the USA, from coast to coast, doctors began seeing strange cases of pneumonia and cancers in gay men they were treating. At the time, still confused by the root cause of these strange infections and deaths, they referred to the virus as GRID (Gay-Related Immune Deficiency). This name was short-lived as the patient pool began to expand to men, women, children, and especially people who had had blood transfusions. By 1982, there was a sense that the disease was blood-related, and it had officially been named AIDS. After rapid studies were performed on AIDS patients, by 1986, the cause of AIDS was identified as the HIV.[34]

The origin of the virus was another matter altogether. In 1985, there was an AIDS-adjacent disease that was found in monkeys in Africa. When the blood of these infected monkeys was analyzed, it was found to be very similar to what was found in AIDS patients. Researchers today believe that the transmission of the disease to humans came from hunters in Cameroon handling monkey meat in the early 1900s. Once the virus was inside of humans, it changed and mutated into what is seen in some viruses today. It passed from person to person via drug use, sexual contact, and general blood exchange (medical or otherwise). The earliest confirmed cases of the virus in humans occurred during 1959–1960.[35] It was from then that it continued to spread. By 2022, the World Health Organization estimates that 85 million people have been infected with HIV and 40 million people have died as a result of the disease.[36]

It is not a stretch of the imagination that a virus that affected predominately more gay men than others was not going to have completely

[33] Dansereau et al., *Pandemic Theology*, 104.

[34] Dansereau et al., *Pandemic Theology*, 106.

[35] Dansereau et al., *Pandemic Theology*, 106–107.

[36] Nikolay Doychinov, World Health Organization https://www.who.int/data/gho/data/themes/hiv-aids#:~:text=Global%20situation%20and%20trends%3A,at%20the%20end%20of%202022 [accessed 5/1/24].

positive theological responses. However, at the beginning of the epidemic, it was largely ignored by religious communities. This is a result of the isolation of the LGBTQIA people from religious spheres during this time period. During the late 1900s, most religious traditions in the USA (specifically) disagreed firmly with the practices of those in the queer community and were not welcoming of them in their institutions. Queer people, as a result, would typically abandon or hide in religious communities. The former meant that they left the religious organization altogether. The latter meant that they would oftentimes pretend to not be living their life and instead conform to the standards of the religious group (if not just for the time they were actively participating).[37]

The loudest theological conclusion that emerged from the HIV/AIDS pandemic was that the virus was a result of two things: risky lifestyles and being gay. The media in the 1980s did not help with this stereotype. HIV/AIDS was seen by some religious groups as being divine retribution for disobeying God's laws. Many people within religious groups saw themselves as immune to the disease because of their self-identified, pious behavior. Also, because queer people often stayed away from religious groups that outright rejected them, there was a view that the HIV/AIDS epidemic was an "out there" problem in relation to the church. In many religious people's minds, it would remain out there as long as the Christian community remained steadfast in their beliefs and conduct.[38] There were some religious groups that did accept the queer community, and they did try to highlight the issues that HIV/AIDS brought, but they were few and far between. They also did not have the microphone that many conservative religious leaders and conservative politicians had when speaking to the general public. According to the World Health Organization over 80-100 million people have been infected with the HIV virus, and 42.3 million people have died from it (as of 2023). It is a virus that we continue to live and die with even today, and it still holds a stigma in 2024. Largely, because of theological judgement.

[37] National Research Council (US) Panel on Monitoring the Social Impact of the AIDS Epidemic; Jonsen AR, Stryker J, editors. Washington (DC): National Academies Press (US); 1993. https://www.ncbi.nlm.nih.gov/books/NBK234566/ [accessed 4/1/24].

[38] National Research Council (US) Panel on Monitoring the Social Impact of the AIDS Epidemic; Jonsen AR, Stryker J, editors. Washington (DC): National Academies Press (US); 1993. https://www.ncbi.nlm.nih.gov/books/NBK234566/ [accessed 4/1/24].

It is sometimes hard to imagine the numbers of deaths in pandemics like the Black Death, Spanish Flu, and (to some degree) HIV/AIDS because they were in a time when smartphones and accurate bookkeeping did not exist. There were also no pictures of the diseases' destruction that you could easily find in a search engine (again to some degree excluding HIV/AIDS). This was not the case for COVID-19. It is not only a phenomenon that plays out in a world that is connected by computers in a way that did not exist for previous pandemics, but it also was politicized and theologized at a level that we have not seen in other pandemics. The rest of the chapters of his book will dig into some of the theological responses to the COVID-19 virus. Using my criteria for bad theology as a guide, I will highlight the way that COVID-19 was weaponized at a time when people needed medical, political, and religious guidance on the topic. While I am sure there are people who did excellent work in these areas during the pandemic, I will not be discussing that here. It pains me to not praise what is praiseworthy, but including them does not befit a book that it titled with the phrase bad theology.

Before we jump into the practical examples of COVID-19 and bad theology, there is a need to set the scene even further. We have discussed the history of pandemics and theology globally, but we will be talking specifically about the USA in our discussion of bad theology. Part of the reasoning behind specifically discussing the USA is that I was living here when I experienced COVID-19, and as a result, I had a front-row seat to the theological mess that was occurring. Also, and perhaps more importantly, the numbers of those infected in the USA are off the charts when compared to other countries that are similar in scope. Deaths, even worse. So, what created this scenario where the virus would have the opportunity to wreck us the way that it did? I believe it was political and social to be sure, but I also hold that it was deeply theological. It was a perfect storm, really. Americans were amazingly equipped to deal with the virus in terms of finances, but poorly equipped when it comes to theology. When examined through a theological lens, we never stood a chance against it.

CHAPTER 5

Prosperity, Premillennialism, Partisanship, and Politicians

> In this respect they had adapted themselves to the very condition of the plague, all the more potent for its mediocrity. None of us was capable any longer of any exalted emotion; all had trite monotonous feelings. 'It's high time it stopped,' people would say, because in time of calamity the obvious thing is to desire its end, and in fact they wanted it to end. But when making such remarks, we felt none of the passionate yearning or fierce resentment of the early phase; we merely voiced one of the few clear ideas that lingered in the twilight of our minds. The furious revolt of the first weeks had given place to vast despondency.... Naturally they retained the attitudes of sadness and suffering, but they had ceased to feel their sting. Indeed, to some, Dr. Rieux among them, this precisely was the most disheartening thing: that the habit of despair is worse than despair itself.[1]

This book looks at bad theology in a time of COVID-19, but it also looks specifically within the context of the United States of America. The reasoning behind this is multipurpose, and predominately it was the geographical area that I am from and have lived for most of my life, but it is also the area where I weathered the pandemic myself. It became a perfect case study in my mind when I looked around and started to unpack all the events that had begun to unfold around me. Horror, disbelief, and anger were all emotions that I felt at any given time, and these emotions were

[1] Camus, *The Plague*, 181.

L. Robinson, *Bad Theology in a Time of COVID*,
https://doi.org/10.1007/978-3-031-75294-0_5

oftentimes the result of bad theology. Accordingly, I am going to give you some background on four unique aspects of the USA that I believe led to over a million deaths from the pandemic. Other comparable nations faired far better than we did in this time period, and I began to sort through all the reasons why I thought that was the case. As I always joke, I am a full-time theologian and a part-time historian, and it is to the unique historical aspects of the USA I turn now. My wager was that aspects of these historical (and sometimes theological) landmarks meant that we had a perfect foundation for the destruction that was to come. These four historical clues, if you will, are: prosperity, premillennialism, partisanship, and politicians.

Prosperity

Prosperity, in theological circles known as the prosperity gospel, is the first historical influence we will examine. The history of this movement, for our purposes, began in the twentieth century in the USA. In the early days, it was not strictly a theological movement but instead was more about manifesting God's blessings (or divine blessings) into your life.

> This thinking took many forms and went by different names, including mindcure, success literature, positive thinking, self-help, and prosperity theology. Mystics, businessmen, Manhattan pastors, and storefront prophets alike sermonized its virtues. This was the core: adherents, acting in accordance with divine principles, relied on their minds to transform thought and speech into heavenly blessings.[2]

Kate Bowler, who I use extensively for this section, is an American historian at Duke University. She begins her discussion about the history of the prosperity gospel with a discussion about some unique features of the American religious landscape. The spiritualist movement in the nineteenth- and twentieth-century USA cannot be underestimated for its influence on both religion and society at large. Often associated with attempts at connecting the supernatural world with the natural (think rituals like séances), it was also used as a means of manifesting supernatural powers through the use of prayer. Religions or religious offshoots like

[2] Kate Bowler, *Blessed: A History of the American Prosperity Gospel* (Oxford: Oxford University Press, 2013), 11.

Christian Science, Free Masonry, and Free Thought were prevalent during this time. There was an idea that the individual human was powerful, and if trained properly, they could connect with something that was divine. Not only connect but also harness some of the power of the supernatural into their own lives. A proponent of this idea, and the founder of Christian Science, was Mary Baker Eddy. Eddy believed that Jesus was sent to earth to save everyone, but instead of this relating to his divine status, salvation occurred through his teaching of right thinking. Eddy thought that illness and death were preventable through this right thinking, if only we knew how to do it correctly.

A rival group to Eddy's Christian Science group was the New Thought offshoot. This group existed in the 1880s and represented a collective of philosophers and thinkers who had a very particular way of understanding the power of the mind. New Thought had three basic principles. The first principle saw humans as being directly connected to God. Bowler calls this a "high anthropology" and "an optimistic theology of human capacity."[3] New Thought also prioritized the spiritual realm over that of the physical. While they admitted that there was a physical world, that physical world was always second in power to the spiritual realm. The spiritual realm, in this way, controlled what happened in the physical world. Finally, there was an emphasis in this group on the idea of positive thinking. God had created the world through thinking, according to New Thought, and as a result, humans were able to create their own worlds through positive thinking. If there was something negative in your life, be that illness, a relationship, or even a job, all of this could be cleared up by positive thinking. You could reshape your own reality in this way. Accordingly, healing was an important aspect of the New Thought thinkers. In 1869, Warren Felt Evans published a book called *The Mental Cure*, which looked to explain that illness comes directly from having negative or wrong thoughts. With a healthy mind, there would be a healthy body, according to Evans.[4] The connection to Christianity in these spiritualist movements, especially in relation to healing, varied greatly. In some groups, the right thinking that was required for healing was taught by Jesus and came from God. In other groups, God provided the means by which right thinking could exist, but humans had to come to terms with harnessing that power on their own.

[3] Bowler, *Blessed*, 14.
[4] Bowler, *Blessed*, 14.

E.W. Kenyon, an evangelist who was an advocate of divine blessings of healing, began spreading the gospel of the New Thought movement. However, he stuck firmly to the importance of Jesus in unlocking the divine power of healing. "Only Christians' rightful use of divine principles could unlock God's treasury of blessings, and Kenyon endeavored to teach them how. He called it 'dominating faith.'"[5] Kenyon's message leaned into the Wesleyan traditions related to accepting Jesus into your heart. Being a Christian and accepting the life, death, resurrection, and message of Jesus meant that you were a new being. Not just new in a metaphorical way, but that your whole self was new. This idea was called "entire sanctification."[6] This type of embodied conversion meant that literally, the person was a new being in their belief in Jesus Christ: mind, body, and soul. As a result of the new self, according to Kenyon, miracles were already accessible because of the sacrifice of Jesus on the cross. So, healing and blessings were not promises for a world to come but instead present in the world we live in here and now.

Theologically, Kenyon believed that God was a spiritual being who created a spiritual world. The physical and the material world were secondary to this spiritual world. When Adam first sinned against God, Satan took over the role of leader for the spiritual beings of the world, also known as the fall. Humans would have remained in this darkly subjugated state if not for Jesus' sacrifice on the cross. Kenyon explained this sacrifice based on the substitutionary theory of the death of Jesus, a theory of reconciliation or atonement that believes that Jesus died as a result of the fall of humanity. In this theory, there had to be a means by which humanity and the divine were able to connect again, despite the sinning nature of the world, and Jesus offered the ultimate substitution for these transgressions (which humanity was helpless to correct on their own).

With this newly found connection, the spiritual beings of the world were once again in God's good graces. As a result, they had dominion over the material and physical world (which were secondary). Jesus went to Hell and dominated the place, and as a result, there is no power that Hell/Satan has over humans who truly believe. "Christians, now unburdened by sin, hovered only a little lower than angels."[7] Kenyon believed that this new status for humans put them very close to a divine status

[5] Bowler, *Blessed*, 15.
[6] Bowler, *Blessed*, 16.
[7] Bowler, *Blessed*, 18.

themselves. Accordingly, he saw believers as having rights to the blessings and healings that God possessed.

New Thought and Kenyon's theology are the foundation of what would develop through the years in the USA as the prosperity gospel. For the sake of this book and its argument, it is vital to understand these theological leanings. Though they evolved and expanded throughout the twentieth century, the central thoughts remained the same in 2020.

> Prosperity teachers, though varying widely in interpretation and focus, agreed on three fundamental ideas. First, healing is God's divine intention for humanity. Second, Jesus' work on the cross earned not only redemption from sin but also deliverance from its penalties: namely, poverty, demonic interference, and sickness. Third, God set up the laws of faith so that believers could access the power of the cross. Believers' primary task was to live into the power of the resurrected Christ by applying faith to their circumstances, measuring their lives and bodies for evidence of spiritual power.[8]

Some notable prosperity gospel ministers in the 1980s and 1990s, who relied on the theology of this healing theology, were Benny Hinn, Don Stewart, Charles Hunter, and Kenneth and Gloria Copeland. These ministers had different views of medicine, but they all noted that God's spiritual power was above the physical and medical powers of humans (including doctors). Some of these healers would align themselves with the medical world in order to further their cause, but others rejected that material world outright. A similarity they share, regardless of one's view of the medical sciences, was the power of prayer. Prayer was emphasized in each of these minister's messages, specifically, in regard to healing.

Another important aspect of healing ministries was sacred objects. "Many faith healers followed the wide spread Pentecostal use of handkerchiefs, cloths, or ribbons to convey healing. For example, Oral Roberts, Marilyn Hickey, and Benny Hinn made such 'points of contact' a staple of their divine healing ministries, asking believers to place an object that had been specifically 'blessed' on the afflicted area."[9] These objects became incredibly important to believers as a manifestation of the spiritual world, ironically, I would add, a material world that was supposed to be secondary to that of the spiritual. Regardless, these objects became a key means of ministry, and income, for many of these ministers. "California revivalist

[8] Bowler, *Blessed*, 141.
[9] Bowler, *Blessed*, 144.

Peter Popoff regularly included pages of instruction on how to use his miracle oil, pennies, or handkerchiefs at ominous moments in the day or night so that believers might exact the greatest result."[10]

In a way, it made sense; it was a means by which lay members of a congregation could feel connected to someone they viewed as having a deep insight into the healing, spiritual world. This was a move away from early New Thought views on the power of the individual and more to the congregational aspects of traditional church; the traditional church where there were leaders and there were followers, and the followers were dependent on the leaders to make their connections for them, at least in cases of grave importance. This point was not lost on those who were selling the holy trinkets to their congregation in twentieth-century USA, and more often than not these ministers would set the objects aside as time went on. There was a notion that despite the ability to make objects blessed, healing ministries also had to make sure they did not fall too far into idolatry of the physical world. They did not want to replace God with objects, blessed or not. This looked a bit too much like Catholicism or Voodooism for many of these ministers, and so the practices of sending out these sacred objects were limited during this historic time period. The real emphasis for healing should be, according to prosperity gospel ministries, right thinking about God's ability to heal, and owning that healing as existing in real life. Thanksgiving at the healing to come is also required.

Perhaps the primary movement that held to these prosperity beliefs are Pentecostals, who adhere to a high view of the spiritual realm and find themselves crossing theological boundaries with those early New Thought members. Pentecostals have the view that because of the death of Jesus, they have the ability to actively participate in divine things in the material world. Pentecostals and those who adhere to the prosperity gospel are not one and the same. That being said, there is a strong influence that the prosperity gospel has on the Pentecostal movement, and this is worth noting when we move forward into the chapter on churches and televangelists.

I want to add a side note here about a subject that I wrestle with in the context of this book. The religious group that self-identifies as Pentecostal is a group that I will talk about a great deal, but it should be noted that it is done so with a great deal of back and forth, theologically speaking. I experienced Pentecostalism in my own family at a very young age, as I had

[10] Bowler, *Blessed*, 145.

a relative who was deeply embedded in this tradition. She passed before the pandemic, but I do wonder what her version of COVID-19 would have looked like. (It should be noted I am using Pentecostalism as a blanket term, and with all terms there are great differences within the movement. It is not a monolith.) While I greatly appreciated her understanding of the closeness of the Holy Spirit and the direct connection she had with God, I was also very struck by how easily some of these Pentecostal groups were manipulated in times of disturbance in their day-to-day life. I will touch on this in the section on televangelists because I do know that a great deal of TV preachers rely on members of this Holy Spirit-heavy group in order to make enormous amounts of money. On the other side of this, I can also see how greatly members of this group find spiritual solace in the preaching of some of these TV preachers, hopefully you can see here the crux.

The Pentecostal movement began in the USA in the twentieth century, and it is deeply embedded in the fabric of the American story. Pentecostals in the USA took their name from the event of Pentecost in the biblical text. This was an event where the Holy Spirit directly interacted with the disciples of Jesus, enabling them to speak in languages that they did not formally know in order to spread the gospel throughout the world. The movement took shape in the USA on January 1, 1901, at Bethel Bible College in Kansas.

> The students believed that the spiritual gifts mentioned in the New Testament which included divine healing of sickness or physical deformity as glossolalia [speaking in tongues], had been restored to the church in the last days before Jesus would return to Earth. This outpouring of the Holy Spirit would serve as the final wake-up call both for unbelievers and for those who claim to be Christians but who had become spiritually indifferent.[11]

According to the students, the supernatural power they now possessed was direct from God, and it was a demonstration that the time for conversion was now. Jesus would return at any moment, and this was proof of that. Pentecostals, much like evangelicals of the time, saw people as needing to have a "born again" experience when they became Christians. The idea was that it needed to not just be a verbal transformation but a holistic

[11] Jon Butler, Grant Wacker and Randall Balmer, *Religion in American Life* (Oxford, Oxford University Press, 2011), 313.

move from non-Christian to Christian. The Pentecostal movement was on board with all of this as well, but additionally said in this born-again experience there would be the addition of "spiritual gifts" up for grabs. The two most prominent forms of spiritual gifts bestowed upon those who were born-again Christians were speaking in tongues and the gift of healing. The Pentecostal movement spread throughout the USA, and when we talk about evangelicals in the text, I will try and specify whether the group in question self-identifies as Pentecostal or not, because this will make a difference in the way they see God's participation in their protection in the world.

Premillennialism

In order to understand the disconnected feeling that some evangelical Americans had towards the global world, and even their local world, you first have to understand the importance of millennialism to Christians in the USA. The theological understanding of millennialism is based on the writings within the book of Revelation. Revelation is a difficult text, one that barely made it into the canon, and conclusions from within its pages have started cults and split denominations. That being said, the idea of millennialism, which is gleaned from Revelation, found a stronghold in the context of the USA. There are various incarnations of millennialism. The three most common understandings of millennialism are A, Pre, and Post. The focus of these theological concepts are the end of the world and what happens during that time. There is a 1000-year reign of Jesus (millennium), and there is judgment, and there are times of tribulations. The differences come in the order that these events occur, as well as the presence (or lack thereof) of humans during these times.

According to the National Association of Evangelicals, out of all the theories of the end of the world, Premillennialism is royalty within the evangelical church.[12] Acknowledging that there are different varieties of this theological belief within the world of Evangelicals, the article states that this view of the end times has made a lasting impression on the church. Ultimately, theology says that according to Revelation, Jesus will return

[12] National Association of Evangelicals, "Premillennialism Reigns in Evangelical Theology" (2011), https://www.nae.org/premillennialism-reigns-in-evangelical-theology/#:~:text="Among%20evangelicals%2C%20the%20most%20popular,varieties%20of%20views%20and%20beliefs [accessed 6/4/24].

and rapture believers up to heaven. There will then be tribulation (tough times), and then there will be another coming of Jesus. After that is the 1000-year reign and then a final judgment. John Darby, a British/Irish Bible teacher made the concept of the rapture popular in the 1830s, and it traveled across the ocean into the Scofield Bible of 1909.

In modern times, and perhaps for my readers now, the rapture-based understanding of the end of times became popular via the *Left Behind* series that was published between 1996 and 2007.[13] The *Left Behind* series struck a chord with evangelicals in the USA. Over the course of 16 books, Timothy LaHaye and Jerry Jenkins describe the state of the world after the biblically predicted rapture has occurred on earth. Those who are left behind, for lack of a better phrase, wrestle with their current state. Many events come to pass including the election of world leaders as well as plagues, disease, and war. A band of heroes gather together to try and tell the world about what has happened, and so it goes. At the heart of *Left Behind*, and indeed, the heart of premillennialism for the sake of this project, is that this world is not our final destination. It is something of a holding pattern for Christians in the grand scheme of life and death and end things. As a result, we are forever waiting on something better to come along. Forever, waiting for Jesus to come and sweep us up into our real home. According to the National Association of Evangelicals, around 65% of self-identified evangelical leaders say that they adhere to a premillennialism theology.

That is a significant number indeed, but it is important to know that this adherence to premillennialism was not always the case for American evangelicals. In the nineteenth century, after the rise of evangelical fervor via the Second Great Awakening, those who considered themselves evangelicals focused on social progress. They were building schools and orphanages, launching anti-slavery campaigns and setting up means by which the poor would thrive. "What animated their efforts was the conviction that they could reform society according to the norms of godliness and thereby bring about the Kingdom of God here on earth-and more

[13] National Association of Evangelicals, "Premillennialism Reigns in Evangelical Theology" (2011), https://www.nae.org/premillennialism-reigns-in-evangelical-theology/#:~:text="Among%20evangelicals%2C%20the%20most%20popular,varieties%20of%20views%20and%20beliefs [accessed 6/4/24].

particularly, here in America."[14] This view on millennialism, known as post-millennialism, saw that there was a role for humans to play in bringing about the end times. The reign of Jesus on earth was predicated on the world being made right for his return, hence the social reforms that were the focus of evangelical theology during this time.

The shift from post to premillennialism within evangelical circles happened in a post-civil war period. The nation was divided, and the death toll from a war that saw brother fighting brother created a world that was less than ideal. The thought that Americans were perfecting their society for the return of Jesus felt far out of reach in this time period. As a result, evangelicals begin to listen more closely to the ideas of John Darby. Maybe, Jesus would return to the world *just as it is* in order to take his people into heaven. Then, all that would happen after would happen, but it would matter little because Christians would be gone. "The consequences of Darby's premillennialism (Jesus would return before the millennium) was to absolve evangelicals of responsibility for addressing social ills. If Jesus was going to return at any moment, why bother with making this world a better place?"[15] Herein lies the problem with the contemporary adherence to this theology. It creates both an isolationist and nonurgent approach to the social ills of the world. For *us*, it does not matter what happens *out there* because Jesus is due to come back soon anyway. The focus in this theological turn is on the individual, and individual salvation, so humans need to worry less about the card they have been dealt in life and more about their personal relationship with Jesus. Evangelicals found the sense of urgency in this theology. Jesus is coming soon was an incredibly effective way of converting people to the faith. Fear is a powerful tool; fear of the forever afterlife is even more powerful.

So, what does this have to do with the bad theology in the USA in regard to COVID-19? Evangelical leaders, in record numbers, still adhere to this theology, and they consequently preach it to their congregants. When presented with premillennial theology and COVID-19, there is a natural response that this whole thing is just not that big of a deal. When a theology leads you to have a primary focus of leaving the planet by any

[14] Randall Balmer, "Conspiracy Theories, Apocalyptic Rhetoric, and the Evangelical Embrace of Premillennialism," in *Sojourners* (April 17, 2020), https://sojo.net/articles/how-did-we-get-here/conspiracy-theories-apocalyptic-rhetoric-and-evangelical-embrace [Accessed 6/4/24].

[15] Balmer, "Conspiracy Theories, Apocalyptic Rhetoric, and the Evangelical Embrace of Premillennialism."

means necessary, the planet is of little consequence. This is not to say that evangelicals who adhere to premillennialism are callous or uncaring people. This is simply to say that premillennialism and its focus on the individual, individual salvation, and leaving this world behind mean that the world is secondary. Any interference from the world (government) to the individual, like church closures or masking, was seen as not only unnecessary but also an overreach. Unnecessary in the sense that Jesus was coming soon, and the individual needed to get right before then. An overreach because the goal of premillennials is not to make the world a better place but to simply be ready. Being ready to leave was more important than cultivating a life of staying on planet earth.

Partisanship

The next P that I have argued influenced our high death count in the USA is not theological in nature, necessarily. That P is partisanship. One has only to watch the musical Hamilton, or read a history text, to see that the founding fathers were keen on avoiding some of the mistakes they saw from their home countries. Religion played into their decision making, and so did partisanship. The checks and balances that we see in the founding documents (greatly influenced by Enlightenment thinker John Locke) was set up in order to prevent one political group from gaining too much power over others. In theory, and I say that with deep emphasis, the country was supposed to move from one political party to the next with a peaceful exchange of power. This was to prevent a dictatorship, to prevent a leader that never left office, and to make sure that whoever was in office was adhering to the founding documents for the good of all people in the country. The goal was to keep the country healthy, happy, and above all united. So, in other words, though partisanship was inevitable with individual rights, it did not have to be what divided or dictated the nation for long stretches of time. That was the goal at least.

Kristen Kobes Du Mez, Professor of History at Calvin University, wrote a book that I highly recommend on the subject of partisanship: *Jesus and John Wayne*.[16] In this text, she traces the history of politics in the USA from the 1900s to the elections of 2016 and 2020. At the heart of her argument about partisanship in the USA is the idea that there is a bloc of Americans who have always searched for some mythological past where

[16] Kristen Kobes Du Mez, *Jesus and John Wayne* (New York: Liveright Publishing, 2021).

things were much better than what they are now. The making great slogan of the Donald Trump campaign was nothing new or original. It had been used many times before by politicians in various forms at various times. Juan M. Floyd-Thomas quotes *New York Times* columnist Charles Blow who said, "Make American Great Again is, in fact an inverted admission of loss-lost primacy, lost privilege, lost prestige."[17] Du Mez takes the conversation further by saying that a certain voting bloc of Americans wants a mythological past, but this past is based on how a privileged group has existed in the USA historically. Any societal shake-ups that see this group "slipping" out of that privileged position cause this voting bloc to grow concerned, and also extremely active in politics.

The voting bloc that Du Mez is referring to is white, American, evangelicals. Evangelicals show up a lot in this book, so I do think it is important that I take a moment and tell you a definition of the movement because it will also be my working definition. According to the National Association of Evangelicals: "To be an evangelical is to uphold the Bible as one's ultimate authority, to confess the centrality of Christ's atonement, to believe in a born-again conversion experience, and to actively spread this good news and reform society accordingly."[18] Historically and globally, this is a solid definition of a distinct Christian movement. I would think that if I presented that definition to evangelicals in my circle, they would happily agree. Du Mez, however, says that the USA version of Evangelicalism has these aspects, but has added other areas in which they define themselves. According to Du Mez:

> For conservative white evangelicals, the 'good news' of the Christian gospel has become inextricably linked to a staunch commitment to patriarchal authority, gender difference, and Christian nationalism, and all of these are intertwined with white racial identity. Many Americans who now identify as evangelicals are identifying with this operational theology-one that is Republican in its politics and traditionalists in its values. This God-and-country faith is championed by those who regularly attend evangelical churches, and by those who do not. It creates affinities across denominational, regional, and socioeconomic differences, even as it divides Americans-and American Christians-into those who embrace these values, and those

[17] Charles Blow in Juan M. Floyd-Thomas "Deep in the Heart of Texas" in *Religion, Race, and COVID-19* ed. by Stacey M. Floyd-Thomas (New York: New York University Press, 2022), 199.

[18] Du Mez, *Jesus and John Wayne*, 5.

> who do not. In this way, conservative, white evangelicalism has become a polarizing force in American politics and society.[19]

This is an American cultural appropriation of the theology that underpins evangelicalism, but in the USA, it has become one and the same.

This voting bloc, movement, or religious group (I will use all three in my descriptions) became key in the various time periods in American history, whereby partisanship has become particularly obvious. One such time period was the late 1940s, and the rise of a young evangelist from North Carolina, Billy Graham. Graham began his ministry preaching a message of traditional values, especially in relation to the home. The enemy of the day was communism, and Graham was convinced that the best way to battle communism was through the stability of the American home. At this time period, it was not a particularly controversial topic of conversation, but the times were set to change, and quickly. Graham was a lifelong Democrat and a Southern Baptist to boot. The partisanship was not drawn in the sand like it is now. The catalyst of this move of southern, white, conservative, Evangelicals to the Republican Party was spurred on by the civil rights movement, the war in Vietnam, and "traditional" values.

The civil rights movement was a tough pill to swallow for many white Americans. There was a re-telling of their long-held history that was taking place, and it was not going over well with some groups in the USA. The civil rights movement is known for helping African Americans gain rights, but it was also a time period when white Americans were forced to look at the history of the nation through a realistic (and not mythological) lens. There was a shift happening in the evangelical world. This shift was predominately based on the way the civil rights movement was viewed. For many northern evangelicals, there was cautious support for the movement. Those in the south had far different views though, generally speaking.

The slight support southern evangelicals had for the civil rights movement shifted when the Civil Rights Act of 1964 was passed. Alongside the passing of the act, the civil rights movement had taken to the streets. Civil disobedience was becoming increasingly common, especially in the South, and this caused many evangelicals to shy away from supporting their

[19] Du Mez, Jesus and John Wayne, 6–7. It is worth noting in this same discussion Du Mez notes that only 25% of African Americans identify as evangelical. She goes on to say this can be attributed to that title being associated as a "white religious brand."

fellow citizens in their fight for equality. Even Billy Graham removed himself from the civil rights narrative. According to Du Mez: "Many evangelicals too, found it hard to accept that the sin of racism ran deep through the nation's history. To concede this seemed unpatriotic. Having embraced the idea of America as a 'Christian nation,' it was hard to accept a critique of the nation as fundamental as that advanced by the civil rights movement."[20]

Another narrative that was prevalent throughout this defensive time period was that of the need for masculine leadership, especially among evangelical Christians. This does tie back to the 1940s/50s and the idea of the need for a hierarchy in the home, but in light of the civil rights movement, there was a desire by some for masculine leadership that would dispel feelings of inferiority that pulsed through the white American public at the time. Someone needed to rise up and tell guilty-feeling Americans that the USA was truly great and also that white Americans were truly great. Something had to contradict the civil rights narrative, no matter how true it was. To add insult to clear injury, there were mass protests against the war in Vietnam, which many in the nation thought was unethical and unnecessary. For a generation who had, in their eyes, defended the world against evils like Hitler and communism, it was unimaginable that young people would protest the actions of troops overseas. This was, again in the eyes of the "Greatest Generation," a direct violation of what it meant to be American, to be patriotic. It was one thing to criticize a government but another to criticize military actions abroad. White, evangelicals were on the defensive about their country and their very selves, and American politics would learn that this defensive position is where this voting bloc most thrived.

The answer to their masculine leadership dilemma came via the campaign of Barry Goldwater in 1964. Goldwater was running against Democrat Lyndon B. Johnson, and he managed to rally a surprising number of those who identified as evangelicals, specifically aggrieved evangelicals of the time. "Goldwater seemed the perfect antidote to [John F.] Kennedy, and conservative evangelicals were drawn to his hard-edged, bombastic style, and to the 'cowboy conservatism' he embodied."[21] Goldwater held something he called the "Freedom Forum" in California, which was a campaign rally of sorts. On the advertisement for the Forum,

[20] Du Mez, *Jesus and John Wayne*, 38.
[21] Du Mez, *Jesus and John Wayne*, 40.

it said, "Voices of strong men ... this is the sound of freedom"[22] alongside a picture of Goldwater. Goldwater would lose the election by a landslide, but when people discuss the turn of evangelicals to the Republican Party, this is a very clear flag-in-the-sand moment.

If Goldwater put his toe in the water in attempts to woe evangelicals to his cause, Richard Nixon cannonballed. "In 1968, Richard Nixon knew that conservative evangelicals could hold the key to his victory. A lapsed Quaker, Nixon wasn't a particularly religious man, but he understood that anticommunism abroad and 'moral values' and 'law and order' politics at home could woo the coalescing voting bloc."[23] Nixon was extremely strategic in his campaign, and he knew exactly who he needed to get on his side in order to win. His "southern strategy" attempted to move historically democrat southerners to his cause in the wake of measures underway to desegregate. By appealing to the idea of the state's rights to make decisions in the wake of civil rights legislation, Nixon was able to get white southerners to follow him to the voting booth. The South had moved firmly into the Republican Party, and it would not go back. This bloc, along with the evangelical bloc, meant that Nixon was able to win in 1968. Partisanship had reared its ugly head in the wake of societal change, but it was not a trend that looked like it was going to end with Nixon, or because of him.

The scandal of Watergate and the subsequent downfall of Nixon as a result could have been a swift end to this extreme version of partisanship. The Republican Party was wounded, but by no means defeated. They knew they needed another person that they could mold to their image and sell to the USA. This person came by way of Ronald Reagan, former actor and governor of California. Reagan was perhaps not your typical conservative, but he had the image that the party wanted at the time. Increasingly, discussions of traditional family values masked a movement to backtrack any accomplishments for gender and sexuality progress that occurred in the 1960s.

A form of hypermasculinity was taking over the USA, and Reagan embodied this vision. His opponent in the 1980 election was Jimmy Carter. Many within the Republican Party had branded Carter as not being assertive or masculine enough and further promoted Reagan as the answer to that problem. Reagan also promoted the idea of state's rights,

[22] Du Mez, *Jesus and John Wayne*, 41.
[23] Du Mez, *Jesus and John Wayne*, 44.

small government, and law and order policies. These were all thinly veiled messages that the party hoped would appeal to white voters. The lines were drawn as the election drew close.

By the time of Reagan, Democrats were seen by conservatives as being the liberal party, full of atheists, feminists, and African Americans. The Republican Party, by contrast, saw themselves as the party of the patriotic, true Americans (aka white), the working class, and those who believed in state's rights, small government (minus that abortion issue), and traditional family values. Reagan defeated Jimmy Carter, a Southern Baptist peanut farmer from Georgia, by a landslide in 1980. Carter, a professed Christian and southerner, won only 4 states and DC. If ever there was a clear picture of the partisanship that tore the USA apart, it was this election and the issues it entailed. The parties would remain in these positions until the time of the pandemic, and their effects would be felt throughout.

By 2016, not much had shifted in regard to political parties. While evangelical lobbyist groups like Moral Majority and Focus on the Family had decreased in influence, the work was done at this stage. The elections typically ping-ponged back and forth between parties with varying degrees of scathing that happened after a president left office. This all changed with the two-time election of Barack Obama (2008 and 2012). Obama was the first African American president, and he was popular in the country. He also passed legislation, elected judges, and led challenges that resulted in an attempt at wider healthcare coverage (The Affordable Healthcare Act) as well as marriage rights for gay couples (Obergefell vs. Hodges). This double defeat did not sit well at all with the Republican Party, and they once again reflected on how they could speak to a new generation of voters in the USA. "New" in quotes, because in reality, Republicans used similar tactics and talking points that had existed previously. Come to find out, history moves on but does not always take opinions with it.

A particular text that highlighted this continued partisanship within the USA is Arlie Russell Hochschild's book, *Strangers in their Own Land*.[24] Hochschild went through an academic exercise which I think is important at this stage. Instead of creating a further divide in partisanship, she attempted to understand the "other side" in the lead-up to the 2016 election. Hochschild is a sociologist and is from Berkley, California. She is a

[24] Arlie Russell Hochschild, *Stranger in their Own Land* (New York: The New York Press, 2016).

self-proclaimed liberal, but she traveled to the deep south of Louisiana to try and understand the people who were supporting the Republican Party, in their own words. It is very easy to vilify a party; I participated in this exercise at many a family Christmas, so I appreciated very much her analysis. Her thesis is as follows:

> The 1960s and 1970s set off a series of social movements, which to some degree, shuffled the order of those 'waiting in line' and laid down a simmering fire of resentment which was to flame up years later as the Tea Party. During this era a long parade of the underprivileged came forward to talk of their mistreatment-blacks who had fled a Jim Crow South, underpaid Latino field workers, Japanese internment camp victims, ill-treated Native Americans, immigrants from all over. Then came the women's movement. Overburdened at home, restricted to clerical or teaching jobs in the workplace, unsafe from harassment, women renewed their claim to a place in line for the American Dream. Then gays and lesbians spoke out against their oppression. Environmentalists argued the cause of forest animals without forests. The endangered brown pelican, flapping its long, oily wings, had now taken its place in line.[25]

To many people interviewed by Hochschild, the core of their allegiance to the Republican Party was not related to misogyny or racism, but instead was connected to the idea that the party talked directly to them, instead of around them to others. The majority of those interviewed were working-class, white, evangelical Christians, and they felt that they had somehow lost their place in line for the American Dream. Importantly, instead of looking backward at those who stood with them, they longingly looked forward at an ever-increasingly small dot in the distance. Hochschild points out to some of those interviewed that the small dot has been small for many oppressed folks for quite some time, hence the shuffling of the line. That is a difficult fact for many people she spoke to, however, who see themselves as playing by all the rules and working extremely hard for very little in return. Another important aspect of these Southern, white voters was that many of them were children or young adults in the 1960s. They saw the civil rights movement all around them, and many of those interviewed actively supported it. The narrative that emerged out of the movement, however, caused many to reflect on their political leanings. "History was on the side of the civil rights movement. The nation honored its

[25] Hochschild, *Stranger in their Own Land*, 212.

leaders. Southern whites bore the shame, again, even though as one man told me, 'We didn't do those bad things.'"[26]

Disenfranchisement, at any level, leaves citizens vulnerable to a wide variety of political tactics by politicians, Hochschild discovered. White, southern, men in her project would never admit to being victims, but they were beginning to feel the push and pull of a move towards a more equal nation. They were beginning to see the conclusions of many of these social movements by way of, "wage cuts, the dream trap, and the covert dishonor of being the one group everyone thought stood unfairly ahead of the line. Culturally speaking, the entire North had 'cut in' and seemed to move the South to the back of the line."[27] This was not accurate of course, not completely, and again the working-class, white people of the South did not seem to want to confront the reality of the upper, upper class, and the privileges they held. Those people were in place for inspiration, not for condemnation, according to Hochschild's interviews.

Politicians

This "deep story"[28] of line cutting that Hochschild describes is a perfect indication of the final example of partisanship in this section, Donald Trump. There was nothing inherently special about Trump politically, and he certainly rubbed people the wrong way socially, but what he did have was a way of tuning into this deep story. Trump was able to read the room and the feelings of inferiority that many communities in the USA felt after a double Obama term. In his political rallies, he was able to bring together a community that felt as though they were, as the title says, strangers in their own land. They not only felt united through these activities, but they felt exalted as well as empowered. United, exalted, empowered, these were all emotions that many in the USA felt as though they were drained of in the Obama era. And so, Trump found that emotional trigger, and he used it throughout his campaign. This, combined with a feeling of irreverence for the political system, as well as a masculine, wealthy persona, meant that he became not only a darling for the Republican Party but also for white, working-class Southerners (and evangelicals) as a whole.

[26] Hochschild, *Strangers in their Own Land*, 213.
[27] Hochschild, *Strangers in their Own Land*, 215.
[28] Hochschild, *Strangers in their Own Land*, 222.

COVID-19 took partisanship to a new level in the Trump era. In a Gallup article published in May 2020, it became clear that views on the COVID-19 virus (and responses) were being overwhelmingly guided by political views. While the new virus caused chaos across the globe, experts attempted to come up with theories about its origins, protocols about how to contain it, and vaccines to try and quell it. During this scrambling, many views emerged, some of them contradictory in nature, and as a result, the American public began to look to their own political leaders for answers. Then President Trump downplayed many aspects of the virus, and his followers followed suit: "Republicans are, as would be predicted, much more positive than Democrats about the way President Trump and the federal government are handling the virus situation ... Republicans are much less likely than Democrats to report isolating themselves, adhering to social distancing, avoiding public places and wearing masks."[29] I should note that this partisanship was not 100%. I know many amazing Republicans who fought against this, tooth and nail, in order to get the USA healthy again. I salute and appreciate them beyond words, and you know exactly who you are. That being said, the numbers during this time skewed in such a way on key issues that it became increasingly clear that COVID-19 was not only a biological issue but it was also a political issue in the USA.

Once the vaccine rollouts began, again the country was divided: "Republicans are less likely than Democrats to have confidence in scientists, less likely to say that scientists should take an active role in policy debate, and more likely to say that scientists' judgements can be just as biased as others."[30] So, there were clear debates about vaccines in regard to COVID-19, but historically this is not something that is necessarily new in the USA. The environment changed, however, when certain government institutions, and indeed private organizations began requiring either masks, social distancing, or even vaccines. Republicans, historically, have challenged what they see as governmental overreach, so any mandate is not welcome (unless it relates to abortion). There is also a view by many Republicans that the White House has too much power and needs to give

[29] Frank Newport, "The Partisan Gap in Views of the Coronavirus," *Gallup* (May 15, 2020) https://news.gallup.com/opinion/polling-matters/311087/partisan-gap-views-coronavirus.aspx#:~:text=Democrats%20are%20much%20more%20likely,that%20social%20distancing%20saves%20lives. [accessed 5/16/24].

[30] Frank Newport, "The Partisan Gap in Views of the Coronavirus" [accessed 5/16/24].

individual states the power to make decisions for themselves. Hence, the mandates around protection from the virus were met with pushback from many communities. These communities challenged these requirements, and some outright rejected them.

In Trump, and in the deep story, the country was deeply divided. Add COVID-19 to the mix and you have a fracture that may never heal. This was no longer about just voting for a certain party; this was influencing how people were handling their health in the midst of a pandemic.

> Those who cited Trump and his task force and those who cited personal and community networks as their favored COVID-19 news sources are far less likely than those who relied on other source types to have received at least one shot of the vaccine ... 59% of those who relied most on Trump say they have received at least one dose of a COVID-19 vaccine ... The most highly vaccinated groups are comprised of adults who in April 2020 said they relied most on national news outlets and public health organizations and officials for COVID-19 news: 83% and 82% respectively, say they have gotten at least one shot.[31]

Whether Democrat or Republican, the public were relying heavily on external forces to guide them during an unprecedented pandemic. They were also being constantly pulled in political directions, while also actively distrusting the "other side." It was a recipe for disaster, and accordingly, disaster ensued in the USA.

This chapter looked, in many ways, to point out a few of the areas that are unique to the USA in order to show how the pandemic got to the levels it did in our country. These are not all the areas, and you could certainly construct a far more nuanced map of the perfect storm that was 2020. As we move to some specific areas of bad theology in COVID-19, namely church and TV preachers, there is hope that this chapter offered a backdrop to why things may have gone the way they did. Ultimately COVID-19 became not only a biological pandemic, but it also became a social one.

[31] Mark Jurkowitz and Amy Mitchell, "Americans who relied most on Trump for Covid-19 news among least likely to be vaccinated," *Pew Research Center* https://www.pewresearch.org/short-reads/2021/09/23/americans-who-relied-most-on-trump-for-covid-19-news-among-least-likely-to-be-vaccinated/ [accessed 5/16/24].

In the article "Culture Wars and COVID-19 Conduct,"[32] you get a clear picture of the battle lines that were drawn. According to the researchers, the high number of people who died in the USA from the virus was a direct result of partisan culture wars. Those who considered themselves on the politically liberal side of the spectrum were far more likely to show concern about protecting oneself and others from the spread of the virus. Those on the political conservative side felt as though the media was blowing the pandemic out of proportion and felt as though their freedoms were being compromised by an over-reaching government.

This was not just a political issue; however, it was clear by the polls that it was also a religious issue. Those who self-identified as evangelicals were more likely to have a suspicion about the scientific opinions on the virus as well as media portrayals of the pandemic. As a result, they were far more likely to contradict any restrictions put in place such as social distancing, masking, and sanitizing. According to Perry and Grubbs:

> We theorize that divergent behavioral responses to the COVID-19 pandemic were more strongly shaped by a hyper-partisan and ultra-conservative ideology that had already been show to lower American's trust in science and scientific expertise; promote a view of (conservative Christian) Americans as God's chosen, divinely protected people; bind them to siding with Trump, and likely reject information put forth by mainstream news media.[33]

I also agree with Perry and Grubbs here, and through this chapter I have hoped to show exactly what they are claiming in regard to the background of the disaster that was 2020. While it may have seemed that one particular party or one candidate or one incident caused the mass death toll we saw in the USA, but I would argue that this was a disaster a long time in the making. Perry and Whitehead ultimately define this blight on American society as being Christian nationalism. They define it as follows: "an ideology that idealizes and advocates a fusion of American civic life with a particular type of Christian identity and culture."[34] I tend to agree with this as well.

[32] Samuel Perry and Joshua Grubbs, "Culture Wars and COVID-19 Conduct: Christian Nationalism, Religiosity, and American's Behavior During the Coronavirus Pandemic," in *Journal for the Scientific Study of Religion* (2020) 59(3): 405–416.

[33] Perry and Grubbs, "Culture Wars and COVID-19 Conduct," 406.

[34] Perry and Whitehead quoted in Perry and Grubbs "Culture Wars and COVID-19 Conduct," 406.

I would love to do further studies akin to *Strangers in their Own Land*, where I do qualitative research to test out these theories. However, for the sake of time, and also for the sake of the text being out while this is still fresh in our minds, I have decided to look next at two particular case studies of bad theology in COVID-19. These are case studies that continuously showed up in my newsfeed. Daily, I was seeing articles about churches opening/shutting, rebelling against protocol, and refusing to wear masks. I saw pastors becoming internet heroes or villains based on their stances in regard to the virus. TV preachers saw an opportunity and jumped on this train as well. Televangelists were, unsurprisingly, taking financial advantage of the tragedy that ensued. So, as I pondered this book, despite my practical desire to interview and observe at the ready, it seemed there were enough examples of bad theology already at my fingertips. We were inundated with it. And since we had nothing else to do, we sat and watched it on repeat. These are the stories I sat and watched with a slack jaw, for your consideration. Maybe you will be less harsh on them than I, and that is absolutely fair. But for now, I need to share this with my community, so pull up a seat and maybe a wine or two. It is to the churches where we first turn our attention.

CHAPTER 6

Church and Church Leaders

> Yes, the hour has come for serious thought. You fondly imagined it was enough to visit God on Sundays, and thus you could make free of your weekdays. You believed some brief formalities, some bendings of the knee, would recompense Him well enough for your criminal indifference. But God is not mocked. These brief encounters could not sate the fierce hunger of His love. He wished to see you longer and more often; that is His manner of loving and, indeed, it is the only manner of loving. And this is why, wearied of waiting for you to come to Him, he loosed on you this visitation; as He has visited all the cities that offended against Him since the dawn of history. Now you are learning your lesson, the lesson that was learned by Cain and his offspring, by the people of Sodom and Gomorrah, by Job and Pharaoh, by all that hardened their hearts against Him. And like them you have beholding mankind and all creation with new eyes, since the gates of this city closed on you and on the pestilence. Now, at last, you know the hour has struck to bend your thoughts to first and last things.[1]

We probably should have known, with all that resided in our history, that the churches in the USA would respond in a less than unified way in regard to COVID-19. In his book, *The Kingdom, The Power, and The Glory: American Evangelicals In An Age of Extremism*,[2] Tim Alberta

[1] Camus, *The Plague*, 97.

[2] Tim Alberta, *The Kingdom, The Power, And The Glory: American Evangelicals In An Age of Extremism* (New York: Harper Collins, 2023).

L. Robinson, *Bad Theology in a Time of COVID*,
https://doi.org/10.1007/978-3-031-75294-0_6

outlines the history of the relationship between the church (specifically the evangelical church) and the state from the 1960s onwards in the USA, and it is not pretty. Alberta is unique in his particular approach to the topic. He grew up the son of an evangelical preacher, and he also considers himself to be in the evangelical category. The book examines what is happening to evangelicals in the USA from inception to today. The inspiration for the text was the election of Donald Trump, who was overwhelmingly supported by the evangelical voting bloc. Alberta was left stunned and confused by this victory, as he saw Trump as someone who in no way represented the religion he loves so dearly. So, he decided to dig into the history a bit and see if he could trace how the evangelical church ended up in this spot.

He begins his historical analysis by looking at the evangelical preacher and conservative icon, Jerry Falwell. Falwell was born in 1933 in Lynchburg, VA, to a family of people who were not particularly interested in religion, save his mother. She would occasionally force him to go to church, but to say he did not enjoy it was an understatement. That all changed in 1952 when Falwell accepted an altar call and became a "born again" Christian. This would change the course of Falwell's life, as he immediately enrolled at Missouri Bible College to study Christianity, being taught by fundamentalists and segregationists.[3]

Most people would say Falwell was an average preacher, nothing super special there, but what they would all agree upon is that he was a master salesman. This would prove to be what endeared him to many in the conservative world. He started a church, a radio program, and later a TV program, and even a university. Initially, Falwell shirked from political activities and generally avoided engagement with civic life. This ended during the McCarthy era and the civil rights period when Falwell preached a sermon "scolding his colleague, Rev Martin Luther King, Jr., for sullying their profession. The goal of the Church, Falwell decreed, is 'not reformation but transformation,' a fact that certain clergy would do well to recognize."[4] One would think that criticizing King would have put Falwell in a bad position, considering his call to tend to all God's flock. However, being in rural Virginia and preaching to an exclusively white congregation in the 1960s, he was seen as something of a hero. Despite the praise that he received from his congregation and the success of his media empire, he

[3] Alberta, *The Kingdom, The Power, And The Glory*, 54–55.

[4] Alberta, *The Kingdom, The Power, And The Glory*, 56.

was not completely happy with his success. The one issue that irked Falwell is that despite his increasing celebrity, he could not help his flagship Liberty University get off the ground.

Liberty had a couple of things against it from the very beginning. As Falwell was growing in audience on his radio/TV shows and his congregation was increasing daily, there was a missing demographic. Young people. Getting young people of the 1960s and 70s to buy into a school in the country that adhered to strict policies on things like drinking, dancing, and dating was a tough sell indeed. Falwell needed a hook, and he knew it. In 1975, Falwell knew that the bicentennial was approaching, and he started a makeover with Liberty. He changed the colors from green and gold to red, white, and blue. In 1976, Falwell started touring the country under the banner of Liberty University: "Training Champions for Christ." He toured with a choir that would wear patriotic outfits and sing traditional, patriotic songs. The following year, he named his tour, the "I Love America" tour, and visited 112 locations to preach, sing, and advertise his school, of course.[5] Jerry Falwell, Jr. was a teen at this stage, and he would join his father on the road. When asked about this time period for Liberty University he said, "That's when things started to turn around … Nobody wanted to send their kids to Lynchburg. The school needed a national appeal, and that patriotic angle sold a lot of people … It had nothing to do with theology. It was a marketing thing. My dad was appealing to a sense of patriotism that was big in Christianity at that time."[6]

Alberta uses the example of Falwell to set up the framework for his book, which is helpful for the book you are reading as well. It shows a means by which a group of Christians were completely convinced about a specific vision based on their sense of patriotism and the politics of the day. Liberty University was not successful based on Falwell being a good minister or having a good knowledge of scripture. Liberty University was successful once it aligned itself with the fear-mongering politics of the day as well as a keen sense of patriotism (aided with a healthy dose of anti-integration and anti-communist rhetoric). That hit something with the American people that theology alone could not sway. Falwell knew it, and he used it to thrive in his business endeavors.

In the interim years of Liberty University's creation and Falwell's death in 2007, he continued his campaign of culture wars in order to maintain

[5] Alberta, *The Kingdom, The Power, And The Glory*, 58.

[6] Alberta, *The Kingdom, The Power, And The Glory*, 58–59.

his relevance (and that of his school). He created the Moral Majority in 1979, a true signal that for Falwell, politics and religion were forever connected. The Moral Majority's goal was to influence Republican candidates to take on certain social issues that were of importance to the group at the time. Most of these issues related to traditional, conservative values associated with family dynamics, civil rights, sexual orientation and behaviors, abortion, and capitalism as a standard. What started as a means of promoting his university had evolved into a full-fledged movement within conservative Christianity. The Moral Majority saw itself as a means by which the United States might be saved from the evils that were trying to drag it down. These evils were very specific, but the answer as to how to escape them could be quite evasive. One thing that was for sure, however, was that it involved politics and specifically politicians who were tailored to help the cause. Enter Ronald Reagan.

Reagan was a candidate that was fine enough for the Moral Majority. He was handsome, famous, and a politician. A rugged figure that could be molded to their needs. That being said, after two terms as president, Reagan was out and so was the Moral Majority. In 1989, they disbanded, stating that they had done what they had come to do. Essentially, they had restored the very soul of America, and as a result, their services were no longer needed. Despite this, Falwell kept trying to insert himself into the culture wars, as it were, but by the 1990s, the influence of this bloc was waning.

> Falwell, had, by the turn of the century, reduced himself to a caricature, more a punch line than a provocateur. He reacted to actress Ellen DeGeneres's coming out by calling her 'Ellen Degenerate.' He ranted about Tinky Winky, an animated purple creature on the toddler-aged TV show Teletubbies who was supposedly homosexual despite a lack of reproductive organs. He predicted that the Antichrist would be arriving soon and added: 'of course he will be Jewish.' He said the September 11, 2001, terror attacks that killed three thousand people were 'probably deserved' because of how America had turned away from God and blamed, 'the pagans, and the abortionists, and the feminists, and the gays and the lesbians'—as well as the ACLU—for inviting such devastation on our country.[7]

Falwell knew that he was losing touch with the country, and so there is a sense that he was reaching for anything at this stage. Liberty University

[7] Alberta, *The Kingdom, The Power, And The Glory*, 72.

was flailing as well, and there was a feeling that maybe the country was not in a place where it wanted the "saving" of conservative America. Alberta makes the comment that while this may have been the truth, evangelicals in the USA, especially conservative ones, thrive when they are the underdog. Even though they are not actually the underdog but have the perceived notion of being the underdog. Much like the previous rant from Falwell, it appears by the 1980s and 90s, self-identified evangelicals had begun to feel as though they were embroiled in some sort of fight for the identity of the nation. According to Russell Moore, former president of the Ethics and Religious Liberty branch of the Southern Baptist Convention:

> Before the 1980s there were two ways of evangelizing. You could focus on end times prophecy, which a lot of people did; or you could talk about marriage and parenting, using practical advice, talking about how the Church could help your family. But by the nineties, being a real Christian meant voting Republican. And suddenly, the easiest way to reach people, by far, was through political identification.[8]

I bring up the case study of Falwell in the church chapter of this book for a specific reason. Falwell did have his own church amidst all his other endeavors, Thomas Road Baptist Church, in Lynchburg. But that is not the reason I am using his story to frame this chapter. I am starting the chapter with Falwell because he, in many ways, serves as a case study of what happened to the churches during COVID-19. When I bring up prosperity, premillenialism, partisanship, and politics, we see it all in the story of the rise and ultimate fall of the Falwells (for further information about the fall, you can check out Jerry Falwell, Jr's story). The Falwells figured out the formula of the American people in regard to Christianity and politics and, ultimately, the power that combination can weld. They could have written this book in 1990, albeit without the notion a virus was on the horizon. That aside, they would have already known the pattern to follow in order to make sure they remained on top in regard to the church and society in such terrifying times. Did they purposefully manipulate people to their side? I am not one to say, but what I can say is that they were able to tap into something in a particular bloc of humans and, I would argue, they used it to their advantage.

[8] Russell Moore quoted in Alberta, *The Kingdom, The Power, And The Glory*, 95.

One aspect of this pattern is the "persecution sentiment"[9] of conservative, evangelical Christian America. In the years prior to COVID-19, conservative, evangelical America had lived through eight years of an Obama presidency, and those feelings of persecution were creeping back into being. The landscape of the USA changed during Barack Obama's presidency, and it was causing that same sense of despair that existed in the 1980s' conservative, evangelical world.

In 2023, Alberta interviewed the Senior Pastor of First Baptist Church Dallas Texas, Dr. Robert Jeffress on this very topic. Jeffress very much adheres to the belief that Christians in the USA are being oppressed at an increasing rate. He even goes so far as to compare the situation that Christians are facing in the USA to that of Nazi Germany. He compares the current time period in the USA to the years leading up to World War II in relation to the isolation and oppression of Jews. He believes this is what is happening to the USA is a slow marginalization of conservative, evangelicals. At one point he admits, "You sound like a hysterical maniac if you say the government's coming after us, but I believe they are."[10] One concession that Jeffress gives on the topic is in relation to COVID-19. After giving examples of congregations claiming oppression because of vaccine policies or mask requirements he states,

> I've said before, 'You'd better be sure that if you're suffering, you're suffering for righteousness and not for your own stupidity. I do think some of what we've categorized as Christian suffering is not suffering for righteousness. We're supposed to be suffering for doing God's will and what His word prescribes to do, not because government goes against my preferences.[11]

What Jeffress is criticizing here is of importance to the overall chapter. He is criticizing those who feel as though they are suffering from mandates when in fact they are not suffering at all. The illusion of suffering, which Jeffress is speaking about, is almost as important to people during COVID-19 as actual suffering. Is suffering having to stay home or is it not being able to breathe in a hospital bed? Is it being inconvenienced for an hour or so in your day-to-day life or is it my exhausted mother, who is a nurse, who would come home with deep indentations of masks on her face

[9] Alberta, *The Kingdom, The Power, And The Glory*, 120.

[10] Robert Jeffress quoted in Alberta, *The Kingdom, The Power, And The Glory*, 121.

[11] Robert Jeffress quoted in Alberta, *The Kingdom, The Power, And The Glory*, 124.

that would take hours to go away? Many conservative groups did not see it that way, and they felt that the suffering was one and the same. Politicians and religious leaders saw this too. Falwell's story of adopting social and political grievances to further a cause was well known at this stage. Religious freedom at all costs became the calling card that would underpin the church's response to COVID-19, which at this stage in the story, had just touched our shores.

Christians in the USA are typically not unified on many simple theological conclusions, let alone major world events. So, I see myself as being naïve in hoping that on this particular front, we might have been able to come together. In the early rumblings of the pandemic, this hope remained. However, that hope quickly disappeared when I read the following headline in *Newsweek*: "Pastor says God will Protect the U.S. from Coronavirus Because Trump Administration Sided With Life in the Womb."[12]

The pastor in question in this quote is Hank Kunneman, who operates out of Lord of Hosts church in Omaha, Nebraska. This "prophecy" was released in February 2020. At this stage of the pandemic, there had been 15 cases of coronavirus in the USA, and one American had died in China from the virus. It was early days, but people in the USA were beginning to take notice. In an address to his church, Kunneman stated that there was no need to worry about the virus because God was going to rescue the USA from it. Why was God going to save the USA, specifically? The pastor stated very clearly that it was because the country had decided to align itself with the right side of morality, Donald Trump.

The sermon that is the source of this article is rife with political language, and it weaves together a Christian nationalist message that is quite clear upon reflection. At the time, however, it probably sounded like a hopeful message to those who were deeply worried and concerned about a force that was making its way slowly to the USA but was also an invisible threat that no amount of armed forces could combat. In the midst of this concern, he stated:

> Listen to the words that I speak to you at this moment, says the living God. Why do you fear, United States? For I have spoken to you before and I will

[12] Christina Zhao, "Pastor says God will Protect the U.S. from Coronavirus Because Trump Administration Sided With Life in the Womb," *Newsweek* (February 16, 2020) https://www.newsweek.com/pastor-says-god-will-protect-us-coronavirus-because-trump-administration-sided-life-womb-1487583 [accessed on 6/3/23].

> speak to you again, I have extended and opened a window of mercy to this nation at this time. Therefore, the virus that they speak of, the bright prognostication, the diagnosis, the fear, my mercy is the quarantine that shall be greater than what they have spoken to you, United States ... And because of the administration that stands in this land, who honor me, who honor the covenants of your forefathers and of the Constitution. And because they have aligned themselves with Israel and because they have sided on the right side of life-life in the womb, life given outside of the womb-there I give life to this nation and I give mercy ... Do not fear. This virus is the spirit of God.

This "prophecy" is, needless to say, a great example of bad theology in the pandemic. When we analyze this section that was published in *Newsweek*, we can start to see the criteria shining through in neon. The human flourishing element is going to come into play a great deal in this book on COVID-19. I consider a basic tenant of human flourishing to be being alive and also honoring the lives of those who are around us. We have life on earth, and after that, we have the next life, but in terms of human beings flourishing, being holistically healthy feels like a good place to start. In this section of "prophecy," there is a direct link to the virus as the will of God, and at one point God is the virus. If we conclude this as accurate, then God is not interested in human flourishing, or humans being alive. God is a virus that is making its way across the globe and is destroying lives as God goes. People are getting ill, their relatives and medical professionals are getting ill, and people around them are dying as the virus moves its way through communities. Human flourishing it is not.

Self-reflection feels like a moot point when something is a prophecy. This will come up again and again, especially in many of the Pentecostal movements that talk about the virus. This is worth a bit of note about denominational differences. Denominations that have a high emphasis on the Holy Spirit have different understandings of illness and healing, as well as the power of God and Humanity. This is why I put such an emphasis previously on the prosperity gospel and Pentecostalism as a distinct form of Evangelicalism. So, when I am talking about certain aspects of preachers, churches, or evangelists as being bad theology, and they happen to be in a certain denomination, it is important to note that I am not talking about all churches within that denomination as having bad theology. I'm not even talking about individuals who have an understanding of the Holy Spirit as influencing human lives daily as having bad theology. As mentioned previously, on a personal level, I appreciated many aspects of the tradition in relation to eternal hope, unwavering faith, and a holistic connection to God. There are other aspects that I did not appreciate as much, such as reliance on a singular leader as representative of the Holy Spirit, unquestioning belief in healing and well-being, and the financial investments required for some leaders in these traditions. We will dig into more of those as we go.

With that precursor out of the way, I approach the self-reflection aspect of the criteria in relation to this section of "prophecy." Part of the issue with anything that is claiming with authority to be prophecy is that it is very hard to challenge it. This is especially true if a person who is saying such prophecy is someone who speaks with authority, as in the main pastor of a church for example. I would argue, however, that this type of reflection on prophecy is important. No matter what Christian tradition you come from, you should be allowed to question what is being presented to you, prophecy or not. This is especially true if the word that is being given to you seems to call into question aspects of your life that you feel to be very important. It does not mean that sermons or messages cannot challenge one's worldview, but there should be room to discuss the said message with others and to give feedback to the pastor. The one voice on a subject, pastor or leader, can lead to danger, historically speaking.

The criterion that says there is no desire to interact with those outside your own community is prevalent throughout this entire message. There is certainly an us versus them mentality as the United States is name-checked, specifically in the first line. There seems to be little concern for the rest of the world, which is also suffering. The USA is specifically being saved from the virus, at this stage, because of things it is doing specifically. Those things are electing Donald Trump, who is serving to rectify a series of social wrongs that this pastor deems as incorrect. These include many we have discussed as the evangelical "social issue soup", including the pro-Constitution (or aspects I would argue), pro-Israel, and anti-abortion. Because the USA has elected an official that will fight these societal woes, the virus has no claim over the land. The rest of the world is sadly not included in this protection it seems, and neither are those who do not see these societal aspects as being vital to the destruction of a pandemic.

Justice and equality do not play a part in this "prophecy." There is a complete reliance on the supernatural protection of God over the USA. Justice for those outside of the USA or those who do not adhere to the beliefs and actions of the Trump administration do not exist here. Justice for those with concerns outside of the ones listed is also not of importance in this prophecy. This message is for those who are included in the community for which these issues are of grave importance, and those who are not a part of it are excluded from the conversation. Equality is also of no real concern here. Again, there is a feeling that the only ones who matter are those in the group. All are equal, if they adhere to the beliefs that are already stated. This plays into the theology of premillennialism that was mentioned previously in the book. Equality and justice are inherently social issues, and engaging with the social world makes the assumption that people are responsible for making the world a better place. Premillennialists don't adhere to that belief system. The world is temporary, and equality and justice matter within their group, but outside of it is of little to no concern (because Jesus will return soon). That is, of course, unless the social issue falls into the categories that are deemed important by the conservative voting bloc, but only those.

Another early indication of the churches' involvement in the pandemic is via a minister named Ralph Drollinger. Drollinger is a minister who led Bible studies for former president Donald Trump's cabinet. According to the publication *The Intercept*, Drollinger has published several blog posts and Bible studies online that contain his theological understandings of the beginning of the pandemic.[13] Drollinger spews out his own version of partisan religion, the only difference is that this minister had a direct line to top Republican leaders. The lessons he preaches are clothed in conservative ideology, and they represent the conservative social issues soup that will become so prevalent in the later days of the pandemic. They offer a biblical justification for much of the policies of the Trump administration during the early days of the pandemic. Alongside this, Drollinger offers insights into the origins of the virus itself, and the conclusions again show his partisan ideals (in religious language). As the world was coming to grips with the virus making its way towards the USA at a rapid rate, Drollinger had an explanation:

[13] Lee Fang, "Trump Cabinet Bible Teacher Blame Coronavirus Pandemic on God's Wrath-Somehow it Involves China, Gay People, and Environmentalists," in *The Intercept* (March 2020) https://theintercept.com/2020/03/24/trump-cabinet-bible-studies-coronavirus/ [accessed 6/10/24].

> Relative to the coronavirus pandemic crisis, this is not God's abandonment wrath nor his cataclysmic wrath, rather it is sowing and reaping wrath … A biblically astute evaluation of the situation strong suggests that America and other countries of the world are reaping what China has sown due to their leaders' recklessness and lack of candor and transparency.[14]

Alongside what the virus represented in relation to God's wrath, Drollinger offered suggestions as to why the USA was not being openly protected from its potential devastation. In a post online titled "Is God Judging America Today?" Drollinger gives further information in regard to what the USA did in order to sow the wrath of God, as he mentioned previously:

> Neither does he [Drollinger] miss a chance to condemn those who worship the 'religion of environmentalism' and express a 'proclivity toward lesbianism and homosexuality.' These individuals, Drollinger argues … have infiltrated 'high positions in our government, our educational system, or media and our entertainment industry' and are largely responsible for God's consequential wrath on our nation.[15]

Drollinger was not alone in this view that the virus was a consequence of the social advancement of marginalized groups. In Spain, there were several prominent voices in theological circles that stated that the virus was a result of the acceptance of LGBTQIA members of society, and consequently, God's anger at this.[16]

The responses to the COVID-19 pandemic were not uniform among religious groups, it should be noted, but I did want to highlight Drollinger and his theological conclusions. Part of the reason of choosing Drollinger was his closeness to the political parties that were in charge of the US

[14] Ralph Drollinger quoted in Lee Fang, "Trump Cabinet Bible Teacher Blame Coronavirus Pandemic on God's Wrath-Somehow it Involves China, Gay People, and Environmentalists," in *The Intercept* (March 2020) https://theintercept.com/2020/03/24/trump-cabinet-bible-studies-coronavirus/ [accessed 6/10/24].

[15] Lee Fang, "Trump Cabinet Bible Teacher Blame Coronavirus Pandemic on God's Wrath-Somehow it Involves China, Gay People, and Environmentalists," in *The Intercept* (March 2020) https://theintercept.com/2020/03/24/trump-cabinet-bible-studies-coronavirus/ [accessed 6/10/24].

[16] Antonio Montañés Jiménez, "Pentecostal Christianity, Covid-19, and the Digital World" in *The Sociological Review* (May 2021) https://thesociologicalreview.org/magazine/may-2021/digital-social-life/pentecostal-christianity-covid-19-and-the-digital-world/ [accessed 6/10/24].

government in the beginning days of the virus and its spread. In regard the bad theology criteria, it is worth analyzing Drollinger's approach to human flourishing in the first instance. This is a pastor who has a direct line to top leadership, so you would think that the main topic of conversation would be about human flourishing and, indeed, human health and safety. Instead, Drollinger focuses his theological attention on the origins of the virus. But is it theologically important in this instance? This is arguable, I would say. At the very least, it was not the main issue of interest at the moment. The virus was present, and its origins as the representation of the wrath of God did not solve the problem at hand. If there was some form of comfort that Drollinger had, a pastoral moment, that would help with the uneasiness that people felt about the origin of the virus, that could have been a good lead for the quote. That being said, what does Drollinger immediately do? He says the virus is God's wrath, but not just God's wrath outright, it is contingent wrath. The wrath is based on all the social ills that the USA has committed (the fact that the virus is present in other places of the world seems to be a direct result of the "sinning" of the USA—sorry world).

The sinning in question that caused this see-saw shift towards God's wrath is a slew of issues that are of importance to members of the conservative voting bloc in the USA. This is a theology that lacks reflection, for who shall they reflect themselves against when God is on their side? Also, there is an us versus them mentality in the sense that God's wrath is a direct result of the human flourishing of others that are not in the right group, according to Drollinger. It is also based on concerns about the environment that are a hallmark of liberal parties in the USA, so they are also included in the "them" group. Seemingly more pessimistic than his predecessor mentioned previously, Kunneman, Drollinger seems to believe that the world has tilted too far even with Trump in power.

Justice and equality don't play a role in what Drollinger is saying to his Bible study and beyond. One would hope that this would play into some of his preachings to those in charge, but to no avail. One could argue that he is arguing for the justice of those within the conservative party against the agenda he sees existing, but what does that have to do with the global pandemic? Justice for what he views as murder, but again, what does that have to do with the topic at hand?

Blaming swaths of society for the virus and its consequences automatically sets up an unequal system. Saying that God is only on the side of those who are supportive (or not) of certain issues is fairly theological normative in many circles. There has to be an interpretation of the Bible, and it will differ in its conclusions. That being said, there is a difference between personal beliefs and political influence. In this sense, Drollinger is in a position where his personal theological/political conclusions, which I would argue are not his own, are directly influencing those who are in charge. This influence is not equal in nature, and theoretically, that is probably why he was hired in the first place.

As a final word on this pre-pandemic time period, Drollinger and Kunneman's bad theology is less about disagreeing with their personal conclusions, which I do, but it is based on their platform and their influence. They are certainly following the bad theology criteria, but even if you turned a blind eye to that, you could see that these pastors are using their platform to spread their political views to those who are willing to believe anything they say, all the while clothing it in the language of God. And somehow, they both seemingly have a personal connection to God and God's plans for the world in a very specific way. What is, is, in the sense of both of these pastors. Their conclusions diverge, while their tactics are theologically similar. These were two examples of the beginning of bad theology within the church during the pandemic, but they were certainly not the last.

Fast-forward, but not too far. It is still March 2020, but we've moved from the hallowed halls of Capital Hill to that of Life Tabernacle Church (Apostolic Pentecostal) in Baton Rouge, LA. The virus is increasingly real to people in the USA, and state leaders are trying to stop the spread in whatever ways they can. One of the ways that governors are attempting to cull a potential pandemic in the USA is through limiting social gatherings. At this point in the pandemic, the US Center for Disease Control (CDC) had recommended that people limit or completely stop any gatherings of 50 or more people in order to control the spread of the virus. Shortly after, Louisiana Governor John Bel Edwards issued an emergency order that enforced this suggested ruling by the CDC. He banned any public events that had more than 50 people in attendance. This, of course, did not sit well with many churches that had larger memberships, but most could see the benefit of limiting the potential threat to their congregants. Many, but not all. Tony Spell, minister of Life Tabernacle Church, decided to defy the order outright. He held services as per normal, and he even preached against the ruling. Spell estimated that the service that he held after the governor's decision would have been attended by around 300 people. He gave an interview to CNN after the service where he said, "I believe the COVID-19 scare is politically motivated."[17]

Spell's argument was that the church was a place of healing, physically and spiritually. He also saw religious freedom as being key to the decision to hold services as normal. People had the right to worship in the USA, according to freedom of religion in the founding documents, and no government had the right to tell worshipers to stay at home. The USA needed a gathering space to look for healing and prayer. They did not need to hide in their homes, away from the world and away from their community, according to Spell.

Quickly, Spell's defiance of the local mandates drew the attention of authorities. What started as a gathering of his local congregation morphed into Spell bringing buses together to bring in people from the local parishes into his church. After his initial service post mandate, he held a service that had over 1000 people. Spell stated, after this service, "[COVID] is not a concern. The virus, we believe, is politically motivated. We hold our religious rights dear and we are going to assemble no matter what someone says, I had 1,170 in attendance Sunday. We have 27 buses on Sunday picking up people in a five-parish area."[18]

One might initially look at this and say, where is the bad theology? Spell is simply expressing his concern with government mandates, religious freedom, and his belief in the healing power of God. The theology that follows is where we will dig into the actual concerns coming from Louisiana during this time. Spell told his congregants that they were not at risk of COVID-19. He stated specifically that the church was the reason that people were not getting sick. He went so far as to say that handkerchiefs that were handed out at the service were blessed and would prevent illness. Spell goes on to elaborate,

> Our church is a hospital where the sick can come and get healing … cancers are healed here, people are healed of HIV in these services, and we believe that tonight, we're also going to pass out anointed handkerchiefs to people

[17] Tony Spell quoted in Daniel Burke, "Louisiana pastor defies a state order and holds a church service with hundreds of people," *CNN* (March 18, 2020) https://www.cnn.com/2020/03/18/us/louisiana-pastor-coronavirus/index.html [accessed 6/10/24].

[18] Aila Slisco, "Pastor Holds Service with Over 1,000 Parishioners in Defiance of Large-Gathering Ban," Newsweek (March, 18, 2020) https://www.newsweek.com/pastor-holds-service-over-1000-parishoners-defiance-large-gathering-ban-1493113 [accessed 6/11/24].

> who may have a fear, who may have a sickness, and we believe that those anointed handkerchiefs go, that healing virtue is going to go on them as well.[19]

Again, one could argue that there is no real danger in this theological conclusion and that many denominations have the hope of healing in their doctrine. While the article that this quote is from seems to acknowledge this conclusion, the author discusses the problems that can occur from this thinking, using the example of South Korea.

South Korea became notorious for its successful response to COVID-19, but it was not always that way. In the early days of the pandemic, South Korea faced a great deal of criticism for the rapid spread of the disease. The main issue? It appeared this spread was centered on people gathering for church. One particular church, Shincheonji, became what some argue, the epicenter of COVID-19 in South Korea (others argue they were scapegoated). Shincheonji church was seen as being a church on the margins. In a country where 28% are Christians (20% Presbyterian and 8% Catholic), it is clear to see that the apocalyptic leaning church of Shincheonji occupies a minority status (despite claiming several 100,000 members). Many think of Shincheonji as a cult, while others see it as being persecuted because of its minority status. Cult or minority, it served as an early warning sign to people about the dangers of gathering in a pandemic. Members of the church claimed that they were encouraged to come to church even when they were sick. And even others claim that when they did attend church, they were packed together in a small space.

But dangerous behavior aside, why was Shincheonji blamed for the spread of the virus in South Korea? In the first few weeks of the pandemic, the cases in South Korea were low, only about one new case per day in its first month. It is the next stat that is the disturbing part. In the following two weeks, the number of cases jumped from 31 to 6767. Patient 31 came from the Shincheonji church, and it is estimated that of those in the 6767, around 63.5% were tied to the church. This began an intense governmental scrutiny of the church that included an attempt to gain records of members in order to do contact tracing. This is where the church did a series of strange things, including withholding records and continuing services despite the number of infected increasing at a rapid rate. On August 1, 2020, the leader of the church was arrested for falsifying

[19] Slisco, "Pastor Holds Service with Over 1,000 Parishioners in Defiance of Large-Gathering Ban."

information to the government as well as embezzling millions of dollars. The then mayor of Seoul, Park Won-soon sued 12 of the church's leaders for murder. The city where the church resides, Daegu, sued the church for 82.3 million dollars for pandemic spending that the city had to undertake. It would be amiss to say that Shincheonji was the only church that spread the virus, though it was the most successful at it.

> In mid-March, 46 churchgoers became infected after attending the River of Grace Community Church outside of Seoul. Also in mid-March, officials in Gyeonggi province threatened to shut down some 140 churches that had failed to implement preventive measures, following news that Manmin Central Church in Seoul had infected 22 people during a meeting to prepare worship materials for lockdown. South Korea continues to report upticks in coronavirus cases, mostly tied to churches.[20]

With the cautionary tale of South Korea in hand, we return to Louisiana. By April 2020, COVID-19 had visited Tony Spell and his congregation. On April 16, 2020, *The Advocate* published an article stating that a 78-year-old member of the congregation, Harold Orillion, had died from COVID-19. Spell responded to the news of this death from the virus as "a lie."[21] At the same time as the death of Mr. Orillion, the church's lawyer, Jeff Wittenbrink, was also hospitalized with COVID-19. Still in defense mode, the lawyer stated that he had attended many public areas, including church activities, so he was not sure where he had contracted the virus itself. Though, importantly, he listed his public appearances as being where he potentially got the virus, admitting that he was not as careful around people as he should have been.

Spell continued to hold large services at his church, and by April 2020, he was already charged with six violations of CDC orders. He told *CNN* that he was "not breaking the law" and that "If they close every door in this city, then I will close my doors ... You can't say the retailers are

[20] David Volodzko, "South Korea's COVID-19 Church Scapegoat is Fighting Back," *Foreign Policy* (August 19 2020) https://foreignpolicy.com/2020/08/19/south-korea-coronavirus-scapegoat-shincheonji/ [accessed 6/11/24].

[21] David Mitchell, "Coronavirus hits home for defiant Central pastor: church member dies from illness, lawyer in hospital, *The Advocate* (April 16, 2020) https://www.theadvocate.com/baton_rouge/news/coronavirus/coronavirus-hits-home-for-defiant-central-pastor-church-member-dies-from-illness-lawyer-in-hospital/article_0e6e7744-8033-11ea-8755-1347b40f9147.html [accessed 6/11/24].

essential but the church is not. That is a persecution of the faith."[22] This was a common reaction to shutdowns of churches in the early days of the pandemic. Cries of religious persecution as well as government overreach were extremely common. Defiance of the gathering orders was also common among some churches.

It was at moments like this, early on in the pandemic, that we started to see that the restrictions against gatherings, mask mandates, and eventually vaccinations were becoming part of a conservative versus liberal culture war in the USA. What was once seen as preventative measures were now seen as government overreach and religious oppression. And at the very worst, they were seen as some plot from the liberals of the USA to forever change the religious landscape of America away from its "Christian roots."

An article in *The Independent* in April 2020 summarized the consequences of this type of rhetoric.[23] At the time of writing, as many as 30 church leaders were dead from COVID-19. These 30 were from the Church of God in Christ, the largest African American Pentecostal denomination. It was not long after mandates began to multiply across the country that COVID-19 became a means by which conservative leaders in the USA could claim religious oppression under the First Amendment. Churches were deemed as nonessential, which means that they were able to be closed by governmental means. Other entities, some quite controversial, were deemed as being essential (which in all fairness was debatable in some cases).

The closures of churches signaled to some religious groups that the government was trying to eradicate them completely. According to the article, in April 2020, around 20 percent of congregants in the USA said that they were encouraged to continue meeting for in-person services (the majority of this statistic self-identified as evangelical). This means the vast majority of churches followed the orders, and many of those utilized technology to continue having services. And this is an important fact. While I will be talking about bad theology and churches in COVID, it should be noted that the majority of churches were following the rules. There were

[22] Harmeet Kaur, A Louisiana pastor who defies orders and held services has been arrested," *CNN* (April 21, 2020) https://www.cnn.com/2020/04/21/us/louisiana-pastor-tony-spell-arrested-trnd/index.html [accessed June 11, 2024].

[23] Alex Woodward, "'A Phantom Plague': America's Bible Belt played down the pandemic and even cashed in. Now dozens of pastors are dead," in *The Independent* (April 2020) https://www.independent.co.uk/news/world/americas/bible-belt-us-coronavirus-pandemic-pastors-church-a9481226.html [accessed 6/17/24].

certain super spreader events, as they were called, that involved religious people. That being said, there were super spreader events that happened amongst other groups as well.

So, when we mention COVID-19 and churches, I am not saying that they were a core means by which the virus spread at all. What I would argue is that churches should have protected their people at all costs. The churches in question for bad theology could have chosen communication of their decisions about meeting in-person to their congregations with love and a sense of humbleness. They could have offered reflections to their flock about why the leadership decided to go the route they did. They could have mourned with their fellow Christians about the sadness of isolation. And they could have expressed the hope for the future beyond the pandemic. Instead, we had some churches, albeit few, who were plastered all over the news for their blatant disregard for science and governance. This is not justice. It feigns at equality, saying churches should be equal to other places that have been deemed essential. That is an argument, and I will leave it here. But I will also argue that the church is supposed to be set aside as an example to the world, and during this pandemic, that was not the image that was being portrayed by some congregations.

Even the name of *The Independent* article, as salacious as it is trying to be, reflects so poorly on the caring nature of the Christian church: "'A Phantom Plague': America's Bible Belt played down the pandemic and even cashed in. Now dozens of pastors are dead." Many would say, well that is the secular media that is trying to make the church look ridiculous. Ok, I will go with that line of argument. But what did the church do to receive an article title like that? Some downplayed a pandemic, some continued to have church service despite people dying from the virus around them, and some asked for their congregants to give their stimulus checks to the church instead of helping themselves. Debates about masks and vaccines aside, this is irresponsible. It is bad theology, that is to say, if theology is present at all.

What was deemed essential and non-essential was used as a weapon in the USA in the early days of the pandemic. Gun stores and churches were non-essential in some places, abortion clinics were also non-essential in other places (for elective surgeries), as a result, non-essential and essential became political on both sides. Were the designations partisan? I'm sure they were, much like theology being a human construct, so are politics. That being said, the way that people on different sides of the political spectrum used these designations to create fear and suspicion was not needed in a time that was fragile. Not only that, the fact that the churches participated in this weaponizing is again disappointing.

Perhaps one of the most vocal of the essential-ness of the church during the early days of COVID-19 was pastor John MacArthur. In November 2020, the *LA Times* reported on MacArthur's defiance in light of the mandates concerning gatherings. MacArthur is the pastor of the mega church Grace Community Church (GCC) in Sun Valley, California, where he has been the pastor since 1969. When COVID-19 hit the country, MacArthur went on a fact-hunting mission that he believes flies in the face of the governmental attempts at warning people about the pandemic. MacArthur used his platform as a pastor to widely discredit information coming from the government. He continued to hold in-person services despite California locking down, and his congregants largely did not social distance or wear masks. He decreed a statement on his church's website where he attempted to debunk the severity of the virus. In many ways, his arguments are quite compelling. In a statement from the church (which reads largely like MacArthur's talking points), "Christ, not Cesar, is Head of the Church,"[24] they state that the church must stay open, according to the Bible. The issue with using the Bible for the justification of defying the government's mandates is that there are powerful verses in the Bible that talk about respecting authority. Apparently, this is not an issue for the church, as they actively acknowledge the verses in question. They point out that in Romans 13 and 1 Peter 2, there are scriptures that reflect that humans need to obey those in charge, even if their requests seem to not be in line with the beliefs of those being governed. 1 Peter 2:18 advocates slaves obeying their masters, for example (another volume of bad theology is needed here!). In light of these verses, the church document declares that it is completely understandable for people to think that they should obey authority. That being said, here is what *they* say about it:

> However, while civil government is invested with divine authority to rule the state, neither of those texts (nor any other) grants civic rulers jurisdiction over the church. God has established three institutions within human society: the family, the state, and the church. Each institution has a sphere of authority with jurisdictional limits that must be respected. A father's author-

[24] Grace Community Church, "Christ, Not Cesar, is the Head of the Church" (July 2020) https://www.gracechurch.org/news/posts/1988 [accessed 6/17/24].

> ity is limited to his own family. Church leaders' authority (which is delegated to them by Christ) is limited to church matters. And government is specifically tasked with the oversight and protection of civic peace and well-being within the boundaries of a nation or community. *God has not granted civic rulers authority over the doctrine, practice, or polity of the church.* The biblical framework limits the authority of each institution to its specific jurisdiction. The church does not have the right to meddle in the affairs of individual families and ignore parental authority. Parents do not have authority to manage civil matters while circumventing government officials. And similarly, government officials have no right to interfere in ecclesiastical matters in a way that undermines or disregards the God-given authority of pastors and elders.[25]

Theologically, there is a lot to unpack here. The three-tier system is an interesting turn of scripture in order to protect one's own beliefs about the separation of power spheres in the USA. Historically, evangelicals have long fought against the idea of the separation of church and state when it comes to things like prayer in school. In this instance, however, it appears they are embracing this separation or, as it is known in certain circles, "sphere sovereignty."

Sphere sovereignty has many proponents and clearly MacArthur is one of those. There are criticisms of this theological conclusion, especially in relation to how we separate ourselves into little bubbles in society, but it was mainly used in conservative circles as a means of limiting control of the state, mostly, over family and church. There is an issue here with how different "church" spheres interact with one another, or indeed certain non-traditional "family spheres" interact with the church, and what about governmental spheres that are more local than federal, but I theologically digress.

The point in this analysis is that Grace Community Church/MacArthur hang their hat on this theology in order to justify the church remaining open despite governmental mandates to quarantine. They remain steadfast that the government has no right to tell the church what to do in regard to its existence. If I pause here, I think this is an interesting argument if you consider just one benefit the church gets from the state. The fact that churches are non-profits, and that status is given to them by, you guessed it, the state. That does not seem to be a bother to MacArthur in regard to the mixing of spheres, but once again I digress. They also argue that the

[25] Grace Community Church, "Christ, No Cesar, is the Head of the Church."

government is trying to fear monger with stats and numbers about the virus (by 2024 we know the catastrophic numbers, but this was written in 2020).

GCC write with resolute certainty, and they do not appear to interact or reflect with scientists who are trying to figure out the virus, nor churches who have chosen to close their doors. GCC is isolated, though they do feel connected to other churches that are rebelling against authorities. They are presenting an us versus them mentality against people in different spheres, as well as those within their own sphere (church) who do not agree with their decisions. There are no alternative perspectives in this statement, the word of the church is the word on the subject. Also, in one part of the statement, they write that churches should be autonomous in making their own decisions, and in the final part of the statement, they say: "Our prayer is that every faithful congregation will stand with us in obedience to our Lord as Christians have done through the centuries."[26] So churches are free to govern themselves, but "faithful congregations" should stand "in obedience" with the position of their church. There seems to be a pretty clear contradiction here that flies in the face of the spheres' theology. It places church against church, even within the context of the church sphere. It is heavily judgmental against the church's right to self-govern while simultaneously arguing for self-governance away from the state sphere.

The justice/equality is hinted at in the theology of GCC in this statement. Justice for the churches against the state, and equality in how they should be treated as essential entities (GCC would later go on to make a movie called "The Essential Church"). So, it is present in this statement, and I would argue that this is some of the most convincing of their arguments, in honesty. There is a lot of chat about the church needing justice in lieu of the lockdown and mandates. Equality in religious institutions is viewed as something that is not just required by churchgoers in society but something that is needed in wider society. Equality through essential-ness, essentially. There is one aspect missing in this document, however. The thorn in the flesh of many of these churches that remained open during the pandemic, human flourishing.

By November 2020, the *LA Times* reported that members of MacArthur's church were getting sick, but they were not reporting it to

[26] Grace Community Church, "Christ, No Cesar, is the Head of the Church."

authorities. As MacArthur preached, "there is no pandemic"[27] from his pulpit, people were falling ill. Forbes magazine reported that in November 2020, over four million Americans contracted COVID-19. According to the publication, there were 37,172 reported deaths from COVID-19 in November 2020 alone.[28] In that same month, MacArthur focused on the fact that while there were a lot of infections, deaths were not at the same level. He also made comments about the demographics that were most at risk, and how it was a smaller portion of the US population. All that can be true, but what can also be true is that MacArthur was putting people at risk, claiming there was no pandemic, and not following any protocol for trying to mitigate what was happening, and there were consequences. MacArthur would eventually admit that some people had contracted the virus, but there was no proof that it came from the church, which is fair. That being said, as the stories began to trickle out, there were confirmations that the church failed to take any type of measures to prevent the contraction. Was it an outbreak? Probably not numerically at this stage, but someone had died, and others were sick, and the church was not setting them up for success in that regard.

In August 2021, MacArthur finally admitted that COVID-19 had actually spread through the church the previous winter. He even went so far as to say that his wife and he had COVID-19 in the previous December. According to *The Roy's Report*: "Meanwhile, MacArthur was out for three weekends without further explanation. When he returned to the pulpit Jan. 17, he struggled to clear his throat and catch his breath, and said, pointing to his chest, 'It's in there still, so, you're going to get it, later this morning.'"[29]

While he now was acknowledging outbreaks of the virus, he stood firm in the fact that no one could prove that they got the virus from church

[27] Jaclyn Cosgrove, "LA megachurch pastor mocks pandemic health orders, even as church members fall ill," LA Times (November 2020) https://www.latimes.com/california/story/2020-11-08/la-pastor-mocks-covid-19-rules-church-members-ill [accessed 6/17/24].

[28] Tommy Beer, "November's Grim Covid-19 Totals: More Than 4.3 Million infections and 37,000 Americans Killed," *Forbes* (December 2020) https://www.forbes.com/sites/tommybeer/2020/12/01/novembers-grim-covid-19-totals-more-than-43-million-infections-and-37000-americans-killed/ [accessed 6/17/24].

[29] Sarah Einselen, "John MacArthur Admits Prior Church COVID Outbreak, Own Illness," *The Roy's Report* (August 2021) https://julieroys.com/john-macarthur-church-covid-outbreak/ [accessed 6/17/24].

(despite the quote from above). That is true in theory, and is indeed true for many institutions that wanted to claim immunity, pardon the pun, from retribution of authorities in light of outbreaks. That being said, members at the church got COVID-19 at a rapid rate that winter, and with little attempt to prevent the virus, it spread among members. In fact, at one stage, members reported to *The Roys Report* that they were discouraged from reporting when they were ill to authorities. They also stated that they feared talking about the outbreak at GCC for fear of what might happen.[30] One such person was a former student of a seminary that met at GCC. The student said that the school followed no COVID-19 protocols and anyone who tried to social distance or wear a mask was openly mocked. In January, a fellow student in their sixties died after contracting the virus. A staff member, Phil Johnson, also confirmed there was an outbreak in a Bible study among the church's Filipino ministry.

The visceral anger response that I have seeing a minister saying that others will get the virus next because he still has it, while preaching from the pulpit, cannot be denied. I was aghast at many points of MacArthur's response to COVID-19, but I genuinely tried to give certain concessions, despite my disagreements. But when we are talking about bad theology, and you have a minister who is, at the very least, talking about the fact he is still contagious to his congregation is inexcusable. If we use the criteria, human flourishing is completely absent from this display. There is absolutely no desire for justice or equality in this situation, at least at an individual, human level. I would argue that MacArthur was so focused on the justice and the equality of the institution of the church that he completely ignored the justice and equality of his flock. I'd argue they were pawns in a game of proving him right in the eyes of the law. The virus was ravaging his congregation and he did not report it for fear of consequence, and I would argue ridicule. His members were too scared to say what was happening in the church, and people were dying. Struggling to breathe and saying you're next. What would Jesus say? I certainly know what I would say, and it is not for polite company.

Coming back to Tim Alberta's book, he made a point to visit several churches in the midst of, but especially after the height of, the pandemic. A church that Alberta visits and analyzes is Greg Locke's Global Vision Bible Church in Mount Juliet, Tennessee. Locke is not a name that is as well known as the likes of Jerry Falwell or the like. He made somewhat of

[30] Einselen, "John MacArthur Admits Prior Church COVID Outbreak, Own Illness."

a name for himself in 2016 after posting a video of himself in Target, attacking their policies on gender and bathrooms. The video went viral, it was a fertile time period for culture war consumption, and he swiftly became a poster child for a bloc of the conservative, evangelical community.

Locke quickly saw that aligning himself with other "religious celebrities"[31] boosted his image as a fighter for the conservative cause. Global Vision grew exponentially, and Locke found himself needing a new building because of the surge in popularity. The day that Alberta visited Locke's church, in the aftermath of the height of COVID-19, the church was packed. There was a sign outside the church that declares in bold letters, "This is a mask free church campus."[32] The guest speaker for the day was actor John Schneider, who played Bo Duke on the TV show, *The Dukes of Hazzard*. Alberta describes Locke's sermon in detail. The subject of the talk was based in the Hebrew Texts and focused on the Philistines stealing the Ark of the Covenant from the children of Israel in order to separate them from God, and ultimately destroy them. According to Locke, "The same thing was happening in America today, Locke warned. The enemy-liberals-had devised a plot to separate Christians from God, by weaponizing a fake 'pandemic' to close down the Church. And all too many Christians were content to let it happen."[33]

Alberta commented that at the beginning of the church service, Locke had likened the turnout of the worship service to that of a Billy Graham revival. Alberta contemplates the question of what Graham would think about this comparison. In the beginning, Graham was comparable to some of the pastors that we have looked at in this study. He adopted certain political positions in relation to anti-communism and civil rights, and he even aligned himself with Richard Nixon for a time. All that being said, by the end of his career, he became increasingly suspicious of politics, and especially the partisanship it creates. He saw himself trying to hug the divide between liberals and conservatives, and he proclaimed his desire to be a pastor for both sides. Alberta argues, despite his beginnings, Graham was different from these celebrity-seeking ministers.

[31] This phrase and "Christian Celebrity" are often used in publications to mark those people in the religious realm who have become relatively known because of their public declarations of faith perspectives. They can also represent people who were already famous via TV/movies and who have declared their religious stances publicly.

[32] Alberta, *The Kingdom, The Power, And The Glory*, 218.

[33] Alberta, *The Kingdom, The Power, And the Glory*, 220.

> Before his death, Graham repented for his early political activism, saying he had 'crossed the line' in ways that harmed his witness for Christ. Still, even in his most unscrupulous moments, Graham was a paragon compared to the self-seekers who would follow him, from the televangelists of the 1970s and '80s all the way to the Ralph Reeds and Greg Lockes of today. There was no foaming, mad-as-hell partisanship to be found at a Graham rally. There were no guns, no calls for violence, no swarms of people dressed-and visibly ready-for combat.[34]

Locke, on the other hand, fancied himself in some cosmic battle for the heart of America. The tool by which Locke would gather his Christian army? Facebook, of course. Whether it was filming in Target, outside of public schools, or heckling legislatures, Locke amassed a following by tapping into whatever social issue was at the top of the pyramid of evangelical oppression on a given day. COVID-19 offered more than enough opportunity to further his campaign.

Prior to COVID-19, Locke was viewed by many in top evangelical circles as a bit of a quack, but that swiftly changed when the virus hit our shores. "When the virus arrived, and the question of shutting down became a defining litmus test for churches nationwide, Locke went from pariah to prophet ... pastors who had defied the government—especially those pastors who made a show of it, then watched attendance double and donations triple."[35] Locke was one of these preachers and refused to shut down Global Vision in the midst of the pandemic. Locke positioned himself as something of a superhero who was here to defend the religious freedom of those who were being oppressed by an overreaching government. He compared himself to the pastors who did shut down their churches in light of safety mandates, and he actively degraded them for their actions. He condemned Christians in America for shirking from their duties as representatives of Christ in the USA. In the midst of all of this, "His following kept increasing and he kept pushing the limits. His viral videos became ever less about Jesus Christ and ever more about Greg Locke: railing against medical authorities, jeering Biden, discrediting vaccines, protesting in D.C. on January 6 ... Suddenly the reward found in loving one's enemies seemed trivial relative to the reward found for in hating them."[36]

[34] Alberta, *The Kingdom, The Power, And the Glory*, 221.
[35] Alberta, *The Kingdom, The Power, And the Glory*, 229.
[36] Alberta, *The Kingdom, The Power, And the Glory*, 224.

When the Delta variant of COVID-19 entered the scene in 2021, there were talks of more shutdowns. Of course, Locke had thoughts about this. He said the variant was not real, and that the vaccine was "sugar water."[37] He told congregants if they wore masks to his church, he would turn them away. He also firmly declared that he would not shut his church in this wave, "they'll be serving Frostys in hell before we shut this place down."[38]

In many ways, it is tough to analyze someone like Locke in regard to bad theology. The main reason is that at this stage in the chapter, any discernible theology has really decreased significantly into a political mess. I may need another book that is dedicated to bad pastoring, regardless of theological content. As per previous pastors in this chapter, Locke is seriously struggling with the human flourishing aspect of his congregation. Let us say that social distancing or vaccines or masks do not help at all, as per his thoughts. What does help? I do not see any real guidance in regard to how his congregants are supposed to live their lives, other than to come to church. Community as "essential" is certainly an argument that was made during the pandemic. That being said, based on Locke's declarations, it appears to be more about "they" better not try and shut our doors or else (who do they think they are), as opposed to, this building is important, this gathering together is important, this worship of our Lord is important, and there are consequences to our community when it is not available, so please consider that in your decisions. Locke became popular with the masses when he was controversial, and so he continued to be. He tapped into a market of people who were feeling paranoid and defensive, and perhaps even a bit lonely in the isolation of the pandemic. Was that the motivation for him keeping his church open? If so, it might be understandable, but that does not appear to be the case. So, human flourishing is debatable here. Unless the human is Greg Locke, of course.

In regard to self-reflection, after the official worship service, Alberta actually did get an interview with Locke, and he is quick to point out that the veil slipped a little at points. Locke did have concerns about his church, and he expressed those in this interview. At the time of the chat between

[37] Kaylin Jorge and Harriett Wallace, "Middle Tennessee Pastor Calls Delta Variant Nonsense, Will Turn Away People Who Wear Masks," *WZTV Nashville*, https://fox17.com/news/local/middle-tennessee-pastor-calls-delta-variant-nonsense-will-turn-away-people-who-wear-masks-covid-19-coronavirus-greg-locke-vanderbilt-hospital-doctor-vaccination-misinformation [accessed 6/20/24].

[38] Jorge and Wallace, "Middle Tennessee Pastor Calls Delta Variant Nonsense, Will Turn Away People Who Wear Masks."

Alberta and Locke, Global Vision was averaging around 2000 attendees a week to church services. In what was perhaps a surprising admission, Locke was concerned that people were coming to his service for the wrong reasons. He lamented the conspiracy theories around Qanon, and how people had brought these conspiracies into the church. They expected Locke to further some of the theories proposed by this underground sect, but Locke was not interested. Despite holding certain views about COVID-19, stolen elections, and child sex-trafficking, he did not see the connection between keyboard warriors debating tales of mysterious messengers and the message of Jesus Christ. Alberta pushed back on Locke on this point, saying it is very possible that people assume the two messages are the same when they hear it coming from their minister each week. Locke conceded this point, "Are there times that it's been perceived that I care more about the kingdom of earth than the kingdom of heaven? Probably. And that was probably my fault. I probably shot myself in the foot and got a little too animated about things."[39] This is an important confession, to be sure, but Alberta is quick to say that Locke was right back to his old ways after the interview. Preaching on all the social and political things that he confessed made him seem as though he cared more about status than souls. Self-reflection without some sort of adjustment based on those admissions? I would say that is not reflection at all.

An us versus them mentality is at the heart of Locke's theology. I do not think he would have nearly the numbers in his church if he had not created a context whereby people felt as though they were perpetually being attacked by the ever-present *them*. As mentioned in previous sections, there is a historical tendency for evangelicals to lean into an oppression narrative, and Global Vision is no exception. Most of his accusations against the government, Biden, the election narrative, and liberals in general create a system by which he is leading the battle into the fight for what is right, against the proverbial them. His entire ministry is based on us versus them (remember that Target video), and it continues to hang on this narrative.

This leads to the isolation of his theology. One could argue that he has attracted so many celebrity friends and so many congregants because he is speaking to a multitude, but I do believe that is not accurate. He is certainly tapping into a similarly minded group in the USA, and the numbers at his church are impressive, but if we look back at the percentage of

[39] Greg Locke quoted in Alberta, *The Kingdom, The Power, And the Glory*, 226.

people in the USA who actually adhered to government mandates, many of these evangelicals, the numbers in his church look small. Fundamentally, Locke and his congregation are isolated, it is why they make the news. If this was a common occurrence, they would not be going viral or making local TV. So, while millions of views on social media or thousands at a church on a Sunday give the impression of acceptance, in many ways it reflects the voyeurism of isolation. Being isolated does not mean that you are small in numbers, necessarily, it means you are separated from a wider body. This, I believe, defines Global Vision.

Fights for justice, like many of the other congregations that reacted badly to the COVID-19 mandates, are entirely internal in nature. While Locke proclaims that his church is working towards achieving justice in the wider world via their pushing back against regulations against gatherings and masks and so on, what they are really doing is achieving a personal sense of justice within their own walls. In my criteria, I said justice will look different depending on the context, so one could argue that they are performing their own acts of justice. I will concede that for all of my examples, but I would also push back and say, does justice need to have a selfless nature to it? Is there an externalization that should be happening? The version of justice that I see in these places is certainly one that is celebrated by those within the community, but it is often lamented by those who are outside of it. Again, this can still be justice, if we think back to fights for justice and equality during the civil rights movement. Some people were excited, and some fought hard against it. That being said, that particular fight for justice was for those within the movement as well as those outside the movement. There was a selfless nature to it. It was externalized beyond the walls of the gathering places of the leaders in the movement. Those within groups like Global Vision might claim they are working for the wider world of evangelicals, but many of those same evangelicals reject their position and their methods. I would also argue that aside from that, their intentions are not inherently selfless. They are self-interested, internalized, and antagonistic, especially Locke and those in leadership. Alberta summarizes it well:

> What binds them together … the scores of other right-wing pastors I'd encountered over the past few years-is that they are now expected to be something more than mere church leaders. They are political handicappers, social commentators, media critics, information gatekeepers. And they have only themselves to blame: It turns out, when a pastor decides that churches

> should do more than just worship God, congregants decide that their pastor should do more than just preach … Pastors already struggle to provide all the answers written down inside their book. In a modern evangelical culture that punishes uncertainty—where weakness is wokeness, where indecision is the wrong decision-asking pastors to provide all the other answers is a recipe for institutional ruin. Because what their congregations crave, more and more, is not so much objective religious instruction but subjective religious justification, a clergy-endorsed rationale for living their lives in a manner that might otherwise feel unbecoming for a Christian.[40]

Is there a desire for equality in this congregation? The extreme nature of the us versus them in this scenario really limits how equal one could be in relation to their fellow human in this context. I am sure Locke, again, sees himself as fighting for some sort of equality in the USA, but then again, is what he is fighting for equality or special treatment? The use of religious freedom as an excuse to ignore government mandates, whatever your view on the veracity of the claim, is asking for an alternative status than other businesses/communities. Now, in COVID-19, this was already taking place with the essential/non-essential status. I would argue that this set up groups of people against one another at its very core. The argument of what is essential and what is not and who decided this is certainly one that needs further examination, but for today, I will say, the churches had a status. They may not have liked it, nor agreed with it, but in the case of Global Vision, they chose to completely ignore it. As I've said, the fight over the status is separate, the fight over what they did with that status is something altogether different. Ignoring governmental decisions happens, but I do not see how this is in any way an argument for equality. If anything, it was an argument for adjustment of status in a system that was already inherently unequal.

I'm aware that up until this point, I have focused on majority white evangelical/Pentecostal churches in my analysis. This is not at all to skirt the troubles that churches with predominately people of color had during this time. Especially, I would add, in the midst of events like the murder of George Floyd. That being said, many of the bad theology issues that I describe in this book are predominantly focused on the white church. The racial concepts of Covid are explored in the book, *Religion, Race, and*

[40] Alberta, *The Kingdom, The Power, And the Glory*, 230–1.

COVID-19: Confronting White Supremacy in the Pandemic,[41] edited by Stacey M. Floyd-Thomas. I can't recommend this book enough, as it helped me to see beyond this narrow world that I was researching. In one chapter in this collection, David Gushee discusses the racial element in relation to adherence to mandates in the USA:

> Throughout the spring of 2020 reports emerged from various parts of the country of churches that were meeting despite temporary government bans on gathering of more than ten people, or were meeting without following current social distancing mandates, or were sending young adults to trips and to camps despite the manifest danger of such events becoming 'super-spreaders.' Every church that I saw in such news accounts can fairly be described as fundamentalist, Pentecostal, or evangelical; almost all were white churches.[42]

And so, it seems to be accurate. By most accounts, predominately black churches in the USA were far more united in their approach to the pandemic. *Christianity Today* published an article titled: "COVID-19 hit Black Churches harder, but they weathered it better,"[43] which I think is an apt summary, from what I have researched. Black churches were disproportionately affected by the pandemic. The article offers several studies that have been conducted to show this problem. One study showed that in May 2020, African Americans accounted for 28% of COVID-19 deaths in New York City. This is despite only representing 22% of the overall population.

A pastor from Jackson, Mississippi, and head of the National Baptist Convention, Jerry Young made the following statement: "I do not know anything that has adversely affected the church as much as COVID has."[44] He added that he did not think that the mental health of the pastors, who were forced to carry the weight of the pandemic and the death of George Floyd, was being taken into account in the aftermath. This disparity in

[41] Stacey M. Floyd-Thomas ed., *Religion, Race, and Covid-19: Confronting White Supremacy in the Pandemic* (New York: New York University Press, 2022).

[42] David Gushee, "Toxic Religion, Toxic Churches, and Toxic Policies," in *Religion, Race, and Covid-19*, 240.

[43] Emily Belz, "Covid-19 hit Black Churches harder, but they weathered it better," *Christianity Today* (September 2023) https://www.christianitytoday.com/news/2023/september/covid-study-pandemic-churches-black-african-american-impact.html [accessed 6/27/24].

[44] Belz, "Covid-19 hit Black Churches harder, but they weathered it better."

infections may be the reason why there was a more unified response to the pandemic mandates that were put into place. According to the *Christianity Today* article about two-thirds of African American congregations had an "extremely positive"[45] response to the health measures that were brought into place in the pandemic. This is compared to only 20% of majority-white congregations who shared that positive response. Black congregations were also far more likely to continue practicing social distancing and masking well after mandates had been lifted, according to the research in the article. This does not mean that there were no struggles for these congregations despite their compliance. As noted, there were still deaths in the churches at a higher rate than others, and getting people to take the vaccine was also a struggle. Also, pastors noted that it has been harder to get people back in the church post-pandemic. Young, when asked about whether he wanted to have in-person services, said he did not feel morally able to tell people to come to services in the midst of the pandemic. He stated: "People would have come because the Pastor says, 'Come.' I made a decision for the people entrusted to my care."[46]

Gushee commented on this interesting comparison between the white churches who defied orders and the black churches that largely complied. He sees this especially in relation to the white, Pentecostal church: "Especially during the early days of the crisis, magical thinking surfaced among some of these same Christians. Especially on the Pentecostal side of American Christianity, occasional examples surfaced of ministers claiming some kinds of supernatural immunity, divine healing power, or miraculously pure HVAC systems in relation to COVID-19."[47] He says this reaction is in stark contrast to the way black churches responded to the news of the pandemic, or even black Pentecostal churches for that matter. The split between white and black Pentecostalism was made especially clear in the pandemic, according to Gushee. He recalls, "White Pentecostals often joined President Trump and their white coreligionists in his politicized and magical-thinking downplaying of the virus. I did not spot any news accounts in the spring or summer of 2020 in which Black-or Hispanic-led Pentecostal (or any other) churches were making magical immunity claims."[48]

[45] Belz, "Covid-19 hit Black Churches harder, but they weathered it better."
[46] Belz, "Covid-19 hit Black Churches harder, but they weathered it better."
[47] Gushee, "Toxic Religion, Toxic Churches, and Toxic Policies," 240.
[48] Gushee, "Toxic Religion, Toxic Churches, and Toxic Policies," 241.

Gushee writes, and I would agree, that white people have an immunity privilege that existed during the pandemic. Because of health care disparities as well as community socioeconomics that hinder needs as basic as transportation to hospitals, there is not the same feeling of urgency in the white communities as that of majority black ones in relation to the virus. This gave many majority-white churches the space to rebel and hang their hat on politics that denied the existence of the pandemic. Gushee concludes: "One wonders if some misbegotten sense of white immunity or even 'white blessing' affected the behaviour of some of the most irresponsible white fundamentalist and evangelical church leaders. It makes one wonder if one aspect of the 'faith' of white Christians is faith in white health supremacy even over the facts of a deadly virus."[49]

COVID-19 in the churches hit close to home for me, which is surprising considering the low number of churches that actively rejected governmental guidance on the subject. I am originally from a tiny town in North Georgia, Ringgold. It is known for being where Dolly Parton got married, and that is about it. In the foothills of Appalachia, it is usually subsumed into the nearby city of Chattanooga, TN. It was in this town that I grew up, a Ringgold Tiger through and through. It shaped me in some ways, Go Dawgs, and warned me in others, segregation is still a very real thing. Ringgold is fairly forgettable, and I think it is ok with that status. So, it was striking when my colleague, friend, fellow theologian, and all-around wonderful human, Kevin Taylor, texted me a link about a COVID-19 outbreak in a church with a message saying, "Isn't this your hometown?"

Catoosa Baptist Tabernacle is in Ringgold, Georgia. In the beginning era of the pandemic, they did shut their doors and resumed services online. This lasted until April 2020, when Georgia Governor Brain Kemp began opening certain businesses. The church decided to reopen at this time, and leaders estimate about one-fourth of the congregation returned to in-person services while the other percentage continued attending remotely. By all accounts because of the decreased numbers, the health protocols were being followed in the congregation. Almost immediately, several families were diagnosed with COVID-19, and the church shut down again. This time it was for an undetermined amount of time. The

[49] Gushee, "Toxic Religion, Toxic Churches, and Toxic Policies," 241.

church made it to national news, and I contemplated why that might be as I read the article in the *Washington Post*.[50]

Critics of the government's attempts to quell the virus might say that it was in the national news because of the desire of the liberal media to scrutinize the Christian church. The majority of Christian churches who were in favor of the rules might say that the story of this small-town church made national news as a warning that the danger of the virus was very real. I am not as pessimistic as the critics, and while I do think there is a desire to sell papers by sensationalizing certain stories- I also think that part of the sensation is seeing that the virus does spread in churches. That the virus is dangerous, and that gathering together can cause sickness to happen. The church offered a message in light of the second closing, and while I don't agree with a great deal of their theology, at least it reads theological. In fact, Pastor Justin Gazaway goes so far as to warn people about the politicization of the virus,

> We have now entered a phase of this disease that is rife with politics. It seems that opinions are split right down the middle as to how we should respond to this virus. COVID-shaming is real. And frankly, that's a shame. Our whole nation is dealing with this together. To try to blame and shame someone who doesn't hold your exact view or method of response doesn't help the matter.[51]

Pastor Gazaway goes on to say that the virus is about our fallenness as human beings, "sin sickness." He pushes back against the idea that God created the virus or that it is a punishment for bad behavior. Instead, he says that humans are in charge of the virus as well as how we respond to the virus. There is a focus here on being proactive and also to get right with Jesus, as we say in Georgia. Again, we differ significantly in our theological and scientific beliefs, but I can tell here that he is trying to explain and contain this virus within the context of his own theological boundaries. He also matched his theology with actions to try and be true to his

[50] Lateshia Beachum, "Two Churches Reclose After Faith Leaders and Congregants Get Coronavirus," *Washington Post* (May 2020), https://www.washingtonpost.com/religion/2020/05/19/two-churches-reclose-after-faith-leaders-congregants-get-coronavirus/ [accessed 6/21/24].

[51] Justin Gazaway, "A Global Response to COVID-19," *Catoosa Baptist Tabernacle Website* https://catoosabaptisttabernacle.com/2020/05/30/a-gospel-response-to-covid19/ [accessed 6/21/24].

congregation. Did he open the church too fast? Maybe, but he also closed it at the sign of distress. I leave this case study for you to analyze and come to the conclusions that you will, but I'd be amiss to not share an example that takes many questions about the push and pull of bad and good theology into consideration.

A final message about churches in COVID-19. These are some examples of churches that defied state decrees on COVID-19, and I hope it has opened conversations about that in relation to bad theology. I tackled the churches first because in many ways it is a much harder endeavor to criticize the decisions of congregations (or leaders in a congregation) than it is to criticize our next topic, televangelists. Televangelists, in many ways, are singular. They represent a ministry, but for the most part, they are a party of one. Churches are a collective of God's people. Usually, a collective of well-meaning people who are trying to figure out a difficult and tiring world. From my analysis of bad theology in COVID-19 in certain congregations, I was careful to highlight the head pastor or leadership as opposed to the people who occupy the pews. Ministry is a calling, and it is an important profession of leading and pastoring human beings in their faith. The common denominator that I see in these churches that decided to not follow protocol is that they seemed to have ministers or leaders who decided that the rules did not apply to them, regardless of what that would mean for their flock. Their desires overcame all else, so in many ways, they were TV preachers without the television. This leads us to the next examples of bad theology in COVID-19.

CHAPTER 7

TV Preachers and Twenty-First-Century Snake Oil

> Moreover, most people, assuming they had not altogether abandoned religious observances, or did not combine them naively with a thoroughly immoral way of living, had replaced normal religious practice by more or less extravagant superstitions. They were readier to wear prophylactic medals of St. Roch than to go to Mass.[1]

I want to start here by giving a history of religious broadcasting in the United States, as it a unique phenomenon to the country.[2] The broadcasting revolution began in 1934 in the USA when the US Congress passed the Communications Act. This act granted the Federal Communication Commission (FCC) the ability to give licenses for people to have access to broadcasting nationally. The idea behind the act was that the radio waves should not be owned by one group or person, and there should be equal opportunity for people to have access to spreading information. One of the only stipulations of the act was that broadcasting stations were required to provide stations and shows that were in the public's "best interest."[3]

[1] Camus, *The Plague*, 221.

[2] This history is based heavily on the work of Dr. William Fore, a PhD from Columbia University and a United Methodist minister who does extensive research into media and religion.

[3] William Fore, "The Unknown History of Televangelism," in *Media Development* (World Association for Christian Communication) (January, 2007) https://www.religion-online.org/article/the-unknown-history-of-televangelism/ [accessed 6/21/24].

L. Robinson, *Bad Theology in a Time of COVID*,
https://doi.org/10.1007/978-3-031-75294-0_7

One of the areas of interest that seemed fairly obvious in 1930s USA was religious programming. At first, licenses were handed out pretty liberally to religious leaders who wanted to go and speak about their faith. This was short-lived, however, as some ministers took advantage of the platform and preached messages against minority groups, like Jews and African Americans. As a result of these controversies, license arrangements were re-evaluated. Radio networks began giving licenses to entities that representing larger groups of religious people, as opposed to individual people. The major groups included were the Council of Catholic Bishops, the Federal Council of Churches (Protestant), and three American, Jewish organizations.[4]

This arrangement worked well during the 1930s and 40s. With the introduction of TV in the 1950s, the platform shifted. The major religious groups were still given space to spread their messages, albeit this time in picture form. What constituted major religious groups widened as well, as the invention of TV made space more readily available. Some radio/TV groups began to give free air space to religious groups, and the FCC rewarded them with credit for their donations, as it were. People could buy time as well, but the media networks were able to pick and choose what they deemed as public interest, and in essence who to sell time to. This meant that religious groups that had messages that were of concern to the broadcasters could be legally excluded from being broadcasted. According to Fore, "evangelical and fundamentalist groups were more or less excluded from this agreement, although the Southern Baptists, Mormons and others were given a modest amount of air time, and some televangelists were able to buy time, mostly on radio and non-network TV stations."[5]

By the 1960s, this free broadcasting agreement was being challenged by conservative groups. The FCC agreed that local broadcasters could sell their time to any group, including religious groups (that maybe had gotten time for free previously). In this new free market, it also meant that stations could not limit or dictate who bought them time. If you had the money to buy it, then you got the time. This meant that there was a scramble by previously excluded groups to get their messages on the air, this time by paying to do so. While this move by the FCC was welcomed by many groups who were happy to pay for time in order to be heard, for

[4] Fore, "The Unknown History of Televangelism."

[5] Fore, "The Unknown History of Televangelism."

other groups, having to pay for airtime was a devastating blow. Many religious organizations had banked on the free time offered by certain broadcasting stations, and with a move towards a more pay-to-play model, these free schemes were not as attractive as they once were. Hence, by the 1970s, 92% of all religious broadcasting was paid by the religious groups themselves. The TV evangelists (televangelists) were firmly in place now, and they would remain so to this day.[6]

By the 1980s, the Reagan administration had deregulated broadcasting, and privatized it to such a degree that the FCC was basically useless. The favor in this generation was with individual capitalism when it came to what was on the airwaves, regardless of the public good. This created a scenario whereby groups were scrambling to assemble as many TV/radio stations under their banner as they could. Stations were sold to the highest bidder, and many religious mega-institutions were happy to oblige. Some televangelists even asked their viewers for money in order to further the purchases of these broadcasting entities. Having the luxury of being tax free because of their religious status, many televangelists create multi-million-dollar empires with the acquisition of these stations. As of 2007, there were 1600 "Christian" radio stations and 250 "Christian" TV stations in the USA. The FCC still exists, and they are required to regulate these stations, but they have their hands tied in this regard. There is a regulation that these stations still broadcast in the vein of public interest, and that they have programming for a wide variety of folks in the nation. This, clearly, is not a reality for these stations. The conservative voice is so powerful in the legislative bodies of the country that these stations go largely unchecked. As a result, they broadcast their brand of religious message ad nauseum, without any type of checks and balances.[7]

The message is varied between these different broadcasters, but only so slightly. The general message is a fairly well-worn story at this stage, at least for anyone who has been forced to listen to these entertainers for any length of time. Generally speaking, the Old and the New Testament are literally true, and literally the word of God. The Jewish people are God's chosen people, and they need to occupy certain lands of the Bible in order to trigger Armageddon. At this time, Jesus will return to the land and "rapture" all of his true followers up to heaven. After the rapture, there will be times of great turmoil and sadness on earth. Following that Jesus

[6] Fore, "The Unknown History of Televangelism."
[7] Fore, "The Unknown History of Televangelism."

will return for the final victory over the land, and a new version of heaven and earth will exist. This message is not new; in fact, we have heard a version of it previously in our discussion of premillennialism. Millennialism is a trope that is used again and again by televangelists, and it is not hard to see why.

This proliferated message of the various forms of millennialism is unique to the American people. You do not see this message to this degree in other parts of the world. According to Dr. Fore, this is a direct result of the influence of the message of the televangelists on the religious landscape of the USA. It is not only a message to attempt and convert souls, it is also a message that is theologically choreographed to garner money and power for these institutions. At the core, this message from the televangelists is about individualism. The collective, and especially the collective in its earthly forms, is of little importance, compared to the individual getting to personal salvation. While Christians in other parts of the world are, perhaps, focusing on social issues concerning poverty and oppression, blocs of American Christians are focused on the world ending. Who needs to concern oneself with the worries of the world when the world will soon end? "Soon" being the important word with televangelists. There must be a sense of urgency in their message. The world will end soon, so we need your money now. We need not worry about the woes of the world, for the world will no longer be here soon. What we do worry about is getting people to the next realm with us, and with Jesus, sooner than later.

This apocalyptic theology is a problem, of course, especially in times of intense trial on earth, like a pandemic, for instance. A time when the global community needs to come together for the health of the collective. There must be an open exchanging of ideas, and of care for one's fellow humans. That being said, if the most important aspect of life is getting yourself and others right with a God that is swiftly approaching revenging God's people on earth, then sickness and petulance of those who "are out there" is really of little consequence to anyone. There are also political and social consequences of this type of thinking, according to Dr. Fore:

> in America there were scores of television evangelists and hundreds of radio preachers on the air, day and night, preaching a bogus religion whose story is a wild tale of the end of the world, and whose values closely resemble the values and worldview of secular America—the values of winning, of wealth, of power, and of being Number One. On the other side of the Atlantic, European audiences were never subjected to this kind of message.

So, there was a difference in the theology that was being continuously broadcasted to the American people as opposed to the rest of the world. This was years and years before the pandemic, of course, but its influence can be seen in the reactions we will examine next in the chapter.

Fore also gives information about the theological conclusion called Dominionism or Reconstructionism. It is an idea upheld by some conservatives and televangelists alike, and it says that the USA is actually a nation that needs to be run by a Christian government. The separation of church and state is bogus in this theology, and people need to accept that America is a Christian nation and always has been. Of course, there is a great deal of historical and indeed theological issues with this theology. For the case of our continued narrative, however, it is important to know that it existed during the pandemic and continues to be perpetuated today. It is with this history we now dig into the way televangelism stayed the same, and pivoted, in the time of a deadly, global pandemic.

If I say the phrase bad theology and televangelists to any number of people on the street, there is one name that will inevitably be mentioned: Jim Bakker. Jim Bakker was born in Michigan in 1940. He knew from a young age that ministry was his passion, and so he enrolled in North Central University, a Pentecostal college. It was at college that he met his future wife, Tammy Faye. The two of them married in 1961, and shortly thereafter they left the college to become full-time missionaries. From the beginning, the Bakkers were a part of the religious broadcasting scene in the USA. They first joined the Christian Broadcasting Network, with Pat Robertson at the helm, hosting a children's show. They moved from there to help found another group that was scooping up media outlets at the time, Trinity Broadcasting Network. After arguments ensued between founders at TBN, the Bakkers left to start their own network.

In 1973, the Bakkers moved to Charlotte, North Carolina, lucky us, to start their own network, Praise the Lord (PTL). By 1974, they had expanded their broadcasting business to a network of religious programming that was national in scope. No quicker had the Bakkers risen to fame than there was a swift fall from grace. In 1979, the FCC began an investigation into Jim Bakker's misuse of funds raised via PTL. Eventually, the FCC would drop the charges, but Bakker was quick to adopt the victim mentality, calling the entire incident a witch hunt. The 1980s served no better for Jim Bakker, as he was accused of misuse of funds, sexual assault, and paying hush money in light of the sexual assault. He agreed to step down from the head of PTL in light of the scandals, and he called a familiar name, Jerry Falwell, Sr., to take his place temporarily. In 1988, Jim Bakker was found guilty of 24 counts of financial fraud. He was sentenced initially to 45 years, but it was later reduced to 8 years. He was eventually released after serving 5 years. In his parole hearings, his lawyer stated that he would stay far away from mixing religion with money in the future.

One thing about people's memories is that they can be severely long in some cases, and painfully short in other cases. By 2003, Jim Bakker was back on the air, this time without his now ex-wife Tammy Faye. He started *The Jim Bakker Show*, a TV show that took a different spin on Christianity than anything on his PTL network. Gone were the promises of the prosperity gospel. Those messages were replaced with something that was far more apocalyptic in nature. Bakker became increasingly concerned with prophecy and messages from the great beyond.

At the height of the pandemic, Bakker began selling something called "The Silver Solution" on air. Bakker brought on a "natural health expert,"[8] Sherrill Sellman, aptly named, to hawk the product. On air, Sellman claimed: "Well, let's say it hasn't been tested on this strain of the coronavirus, but it has been tested on other strains of the coronavirus and has been able to eliminate it within 12 hours … Totally eliminate it. Kills it. Deactivates it."[9] For the low price of $80, four bottles of the solution could be yours. However that probably would not last a long time, as the "experts" encouraged you to apply it liberally all over your body.

It was a story of modern-day snake oil, and while Bakker relied on the witness of a so-called expert to prove the effectiveness of the solution, he still platformed this product on the show bearing his name. The solution was found to be colloidal silver suspended in a liquid. This solution has no known health benefits according to the National Center for Complementary and Integrative Health, a federal scientific research agency. Perhaps one of the biggest side effects of the substance is that it can turn one's skin a strange hue of blue. Needless to say, the state of Missouri where *The Jim Bakker Show* is filmed, immediately sued the show. Jim Bakker and the company settled in court, and they were ordered to issue refunds to all people who had bought the product. They were also ordered to pay

[8] Matthew Schwartz, "Missouri Sues Televangelist Jim Bakker for Selling Fake Coronavirus Cure," *NPR* https://www.npr.org/2020/03/11/814550474/missouri-sues-televangelist-jim-bakker-for-selling-fake-coronavirus-cure [accessed 6/25/24].

[9] Schwartz, "Missouri Sues Televangelist Jim Bakker for Selling Fake Coronavirus Cure."

$156,000 to the state. Bakker never admitted wrongdoing in this case against him, but he did agree to no longer sell the solution to people. Missouri Governor Jay Nixon was horrified by the conclusions of the trial, and he made a public statement that he believed the allegations against Bakker were simply an attempt to get his ministry off the air.[10]

It is almost too easy to take on this instance of bad theology in regard to Jim Bakker and his silver solution. It is so selfish an endeavor that that the idea of human flourishing is not even close to the priority list, let alone on it. Let us imagine, for even a moment, that Bakker really thought the silver solution might actually help people. Why did he not investigate it further himself before putting it on his TV show for all to see? Also, why would he be selling it? If it was some miracle cure, surely there would be some way to fund it for people to have, or at the very least have it at a lower cost than what was being proposed. The other option is we judge Mr. Bakker based on his history of swindling money from folks and his subsequent jail time as a result. Historically, Bakker has not put human flourishing at the top of his priority list, unless that human is Bakker himself.

Self-reflection does not seem to be a strong suit with Bakker, generally speaking. The silver solution debacle was no exception. No sooner had the state settled with Bakker did he get on air to ask for money, again. He guilted his watchers into helping him stay afloat, claiming that without their support he was going to go bankrupt in the midst of the legal woes he was having. One thing he did not do? He never admitted fault for the misguided information about the silver solution. He never confessed that he was not completely sure about the truth behind the medicine he was selling on the show that bore his name.[11] Bakker has yet to confess any wrongdoing despite spending five years in jail, so I would not think that he would start here. For Bakker to reflect and repent for his wrongdoings, purposeful or neglectful, would disintegrate the whole image of the televangelist in the USA. They are supposed to be special, set aside, gaining supernatural knowledge about things that most mortal humans are not privy to. Bakker will not confess to his audience, and quite honestly, he cannot confess if he wants to keep them. He knows this. This is the

[10] Jim Salter, "Jim Bakker, his church settle lawsuit over Covid-19 claims," AP News https://apnews.com/article/jim-bakker-michael-brown-lawsuits-coronavirus-pandemic-arts-and-entertainment-b8ef1bc92d3a6527f717693dbdb4b619 [accessed 6/25/24].

[11] Charles Duncan, "Televangelist who sold fake COVID-19 cure asks viewers for cash to avoid bankruptcy," *The Kansas City Star*, https://www.kansascity.com/news/coronavirus/article242225266.html [accessed 6/25/24].

impossible situation these types of "ministers" put themselves into by claiming to know things that they do not actually know. When they do not know something, people get suspicious, so even when confronted with counter-intelligence, they will deny and deflect. They will not reflect.

We certainly see the us versus them mentality in this narrative. Us is Bakker and those who adhere to his beliefs, them is the state and anyone trying to discredit him. Even the governor got involved and blamed politics for the demise of the silver solution, so we are back to culture wars again. In the case of Jim Bakker and his snake oil, I would argue that the them extends to those to whom he is selling the solution. Us, in this scenario, is Bakker and his cohorts. The audience is only an "us" so long as they are supporting his ministry. The minute they are taking his money or complaining about a product his ministry produced, they get put in the "them" category. The "thems" would require Jim Bakker to reflect on his actions, and so they must be ridiculed and rejected as outsiders. In the worlds of the televangelists, one's world gets smaller as the deceit gets larger, until ultimately the Bakkers of the world are forced to find a new and fresh audience to bring into the club.

This leads directly to the isolated nature of the theology of Bakker and Co. It was a strategic move to go from the prosperity gospel to that of apocalyptic prophecy in Bakker's ministry. He had largely lost his audience of the 1980s because of his scandals with money, so to find a new type of message was good marketing on his part. Moving to more of a prophetic ministry does fit within the framework of televangelism, and it offered a different avenue for Bakker to continue to be on the airwaves. The main issue for the general public, as we have spoken about previously in this book, is that prophecy is inherently isolated. When you are the one who is getting the messages directly from a divine power, it is hard to contradict said message. Who am I to say that the message of the prophet is wrong? For that matter, who is the community to say that the prophet is wrong? The issue here is clear, no one can say that what you are saying is wrong if it is a prophecy from a televangelist. They have a captive audience who are genuinely invested in the prophet being correct. To lose that stability is unheard of, and so it is a semiotic relationship in that way. The audience needs the televangelist to be absolutely, divinely correct. On the flip side, the televangelist needs the audience to not question what is being said. To follow without fuss. It is very hard to break through this form of isolation in theology, and it proves why they are so successful in what they do.

There is no justice in taking money from people for corrupt reasons. There is also no equality in charging people money for fake medicine they may not be able to afford. Shrouding this in the language of the divine does not make it any less unjust and unequal. This is not a healing product, and Bakker was making profits off of the deception. Some form of justice was done by Bakker being forced to take the fake products off the shelf, but it was short-lived, and he was back on the air asking for money once again. This time, using the culture war trope to strike fear in his audience about his impending cancellation. In the televangelist/audience scenario, there is no equality. The whole system is based on the idea that the minister is inherently unequal, and that is what makes them special. That is why viewers tune in, because they have insights that the audience cannot receive. This sets up a scenario where it is very easy for injustice to occur. For people to be taken advantage of, and in the case of the silver solution and Jim Bakker, that is exactly what we saw happen.

The next televangelist on our list is Kenneth Copeland. Copeland was born in 1936 in Texas. Copeland was surrounded by the Pentecostal church early in his upbringing, and he eventually decided to attend Oral Roberts University, a prominent, evangelical university in Oklahoma. He would go on to found Kenneth Copeland Ministries (KCM) in 1967, alongside his wife Gloria.

An important aspect of this particular case study is to emphasize that Copeland focused his ministry on the prosperity gospel, as we have spoken about previously in this book. As a result, there is a high emphasis on the spirit, and the power of the spirit, in his teachings. Additionally, KCM is most notably a part of the "Word of Faith" movement. This movement is essentially a corporate means of propagating the prosperity gospel. It is a collection of pastors and churches that uphold the idea that humans are supposed to be healthy, happy, and wealthy. They believe that since God spoke realities into existence, so can humans, because we are God's creation. Positive speaking will result in positive things in the world. If you speak negativity into the world, that will be the reality that you are faced with. They also believe that if you are suffering it is because you do not have enough faith in the doctrines of prosperity. A central aspect of the movement to televangelists is the belief that if you bless others, you will be blessed as well. More often than not, this blessing is financial, and it goes one way towards the televangelists. There is a reason that many of them drive expensive cars, have mansions and planes, and ultimately go to jail for misappropriation of funds. Word of Faith consider themselves charismatic, which is another group who hold a high view of the Holy Spirit in their day-to-day lives. They began in the same vein as New Thought that we discussed earlier in the book.

Perhaps the most disturbing aspect of the Word of Faith movement, and the one that we will see especially with the televangelists, is the downplaying of the deity of God and the raising up of the deity of humanity. This doctrine is oftentimes referred to as "Little Gods" doctrine, and it upholds the idea that because humanity are God's creation, we are able to share in godly activities. Adam lost that ability through original sin, and we have to reclaim our ability to influence the world in order to do that we had to become Christians, born-again Christians. Thus, the reason Jesus returned to earth was to restore humanity to this god-like status. Some pastors within the Word of Faith movement even equate humanity to the status of Jesus. God also needs permission to interfere in the workings of humanity because of the fall. Therefore, humans must speak and *allow* God to be a part of the going-ons of the world. Not only is this whole movement based on bad theology, it is just bad interpretation at its core. I will let the systematic folks go after the biblical gymnastics that went into this damaging theology, but for now, we just need to know it exists and that many televangelists absolutely live for it. And I would argue, absolutely need it in order to live.

The Copelands adhere to this movement, and indeed the prosperity gospel as a whole. It is estimated that in 2021, Copeland was the richest pastor in the USA, with a net worth of $750 million. He currently resides in a 18,000 square foot house, tax free, that is estimated to be worth around $7 million dollars. When asked about the extravagant house, not to mention the various planes the ministry owns, Copeland replied: "You may think the house is too big. You may think it is too grand. I don't care what you think. I heard from heaven. Glory to God, hallelujah!"[12] Kenneth Copeland ministries still exists and operates out of Fort Worth, Texas.

During COVID-19, Copeland still held in-person ministry, but really focused his attention on those who were at home via his online presence. Copeland's message about COVID-19 is in accordance with the banner of his ministry, the prosperity theology. He preaches to his audience that the virus will be dominated and defeated soon. This destruction of the virus

[12] Mary Jacob, "Kenneth Copeland, wealthiest US pastor, lives on $7m tax-free estate," (December 2021) *New York* Post https://nypost.com/2021/12/17/kenneth-copeland-wealthiest-us-pastor-lives-on-7m-tax-free-estate/ [accessed 6/26/24].

will occur via the prayers of Christians and the power of God. In a now infamous, and ill-advised sermon, Copeland blew forcefully into his camera/audience and declared, "I blow the wind of God on you. You are destroyed forever, and you'll never be back. Thank you, God. Let it happen. Cause it to happen."[13] *The Independent* reported this story, and goes on to say that the previous month Copeland had preached a sermon where he declared that he had "passed judgement" on COVID-19 and that it was "finished." In this sermon, he also said that the US was "healed and well again."[14]

I have mentioned previously that I do have sympathy for aspects of the high spirit traditions. I can see that Copeland is speaking words to divine power in order to have them come to pass. While some would view this as virus denying, which is absolutely fair, I would argue it was Copeland believing and speaking the end of the virus into being, as is according to his tradition. This is where my sympathy ends, however. The article goes on to describe how Copeland encouraged his audience to continue giving to the ministry, even if they lost their jobs. Also that if someone got COVID-19, they could be healed through touching the television, or even showing up in real life to be healed. Finally, he stated in one instance that the virus existed because people had "opened the door" to the virus because of their "displays of hate" against Donald Trump.[15]

The prosperity message is troubling for many reasons, and in terms of my criteria, I would characterize it is as bad theology. Copeland has his own politicized version of this theological conclusion which adds another layer to this bad theology. Like many of the televangelists that we mention in this book, despite the name prosperity gospel, this is not at all the goal of these leaders for their audiences. There is a guise of human flourishing in the sense that you give money or attend services and you will be healed, but all of this flourishing is contingent on something. If the televangelists believe, as they say, that they have eradicated the virus from society, should that not be a message freely given? There should not be strings attached

[13] Alex Woodward, "Coronavirus: Televangelist Kenneth Copeland 'blows wind of God' at Covid-19 to 'destroy' pandemic," *The Independent* (April 2020) https://www.independent.co.uk/news/world/americas/kenneth-copeland-blow-coronavirus-pray-sermon-trump-televangelist-a9448561.html [accessed 6/26/24].

[14] Woodward, "Coronavirus: Televangelist Kenneth Copeland 'blows wind of God' at Covid-19 to 'destroy' pandemic."

[15] Woodward, "Coronavirus: Televangelist Kenneth Copeland 'blows wind of God' at Covid-19 to 'destroy' pandemic."

to a goal of human flourishing. Certainly not demanding your audience give the richest pastor in the USA the last of you and your family's earnings. Also, promising people that they will be healed if they come to your church, or touch a television screen can create a sense of false hope and consequent risky behaviors. This does not lend itself to human flourishing.

Kenneth Copeland is certain of his theology. This is very clear in the way he presents it to his audience. When confronted about his over-the-top lifestyle, he deflects. His response is that God told him that he should live the way he does, so who are we to argue. It is a point, much like prophecy and works of the holy spirit, that are hard to argue. That does not mean, however, that we cannot investigate what he is saying through the lens of bad theology. You are a minister and you are worth $750 million. You are asking people to give their pay checks to you, even if they are in danger of being laid off. And your reflection on all of this is, basically, God said it was ok that I'm this rich. That is no reflection at all.

This leads directly to the lack of desire to interact with those who do not believe as you do. Copeland has not amassed this much wealth and power through reflection and interactions with those who do not believe as he does. In fact, when confronted, he balks at the idea that there is any truth outside that which he has been proclaiming. He goes so far as to say that those who do not agree with him theologically *or* politically are the very reason the virus has been able to be so affective. Televangelists must maintain the us versus them mentality in order to keep their power and money, otherwise what they are saying will be heard for what it really is, manipulation. Instead of a concerned relative or friend, someone who does not agree with Kenneth Copeland must be an enemy. Not just an enemy, but the very cause of the turmoil and strife that we are dealing with in COVID-19. The "them" is who Copeland is fighting against, according to his loyal audience, he is trying to overcome their shortcomings for the betterment of the rest of the world. If only he had the funding to do so.

Copeland probably sees the above-mentioned fight against the virus as being a means of doing justice in the world. I've no doubt he sees himself as a prayer warrior for the good of humanity. That he sees Donald Trump as being a political force of justice for the USA during these trying times. This is all his own prerogative. There is a danger, however, in mixing this idea of justice with a very strict us versus them mentality. If justice can only come through his prophecy and prayer, and it can only come politically through Donald Trump, then anyone who opposes these stances are seen as doing injustice. In fact, he goes so far as to say that the virus is as powerful as it is because people opposed Trump. This leads to the inequality that exists in Kenneth Copeland's ministry.

Prosperity televangelists have faced numerous criticisms historically, not least from me. The sheer amount of wealth that is accumulated by these folks, all in the name of God, is shocking. Week after week they come with the same message, we need your help, but do they? Do they need our help to keep their ministry going or do they need our help to keep themselves living in 18,000-square-foot houses? All the while, their audiences are struggling to keep up with the basics. Theologically, there is no justification that I can see for this behavior. Even if you do have a high view of the power of the Holy Spirit, this type of wealth inequality that exists is bad theology at its core. Also, the power dynamic of someone who justifies said wealth grab as being divine in nature is inherently unequal. There is nothing in the text that suggests that the financial power dynamic between pastor and flock should be that egregious. Mr. Copeland, welcome to the bad theology club.

The next two media personalities will be analyzed together: Marcus Lamb and Irvin Baxter. Marcus Lamb is the founder of Daystar Television Network (1997). As a result of a large donation from Kenneth Copeland, Lamb was able to launch the network with his wife Joni. Daystar operates in the same movement as Copeland and many others, the Word of Faith movement. The programming is ministry- and education-focused, but all through the lens of Word of Faith and its belief system. Daystar has moved into the digital age whereby you see its programming online and on TV. The flagship program, *Ministry Now*, was hosted by both Marcus and Joni Lamb.

In the early 2000s, Daystar was under investigation for, you can probably guess at this stage, financial misdealings in relation to selling broadcasting time for profit. The lawsuit was eventually settled with Daystar agreeing to pay a fine of $17,500 for its failure to comply with its nonprofit status. Daystar, and Lamb specifically, was hit with further controversy in 2010. Marcus admitted to having an affair to his wife Joni. He admitted to the affair and said that Joni had since forgiven him for the transgressions. Marcus and Joni did the media circuit about the affair and the reconciliation. There were a series of harassment charges by employees/former employees that were consequently dropped.

The next big controversy to hit Daystar came by way of COVID-19. Lamb became deeply entrenched in the anti-vax movement that occurred when COVID-19 vaccines were developed and distributed. For a myriad of different reasons, some far more convincing than others, certain groups of people decided to focus their ministries heavily on the dangers of the vaccines. Daystar jumped on this train and hosted famous anti-vaxxers like Robert Kennedy, Jr and Del Bigtree. Having concerns about a new vaccine is one thing, but saying that the vaccine will kill half of the people who take it and that the vaccine contained microchips implanted into humans is conspiracy and ultimately unproven. On December 2, 2021, Marcus Lamb died of COVID-19. Lamb had diabetes, which was not public knowledge at the time, despite much of his anti-vax discussions on air. According to statements from those close to Marcus Lamb, he kept the disease in check and he managed to maintain a healthy lifestyle. His wife Joni said that his "heart just gave out"[16] in the end. He went to the hospital to get oxygen, according to his family, but Joni maintains that despite this he still held fast to his beliefs about the virus that he proclaimed on his show. Marcus' son Jonathan came on the Daystar network and stated that this illness with his father was an attack from the devil. The devil was trying to silence the truth that his father was giving to the rest of the world. The devil clearly was not happy with listeners getting the truth, hence the illness.

Irvin Baxter has a very similar story. Irvine Baxter began his ministry journey when he was 19 years old as a traveling evangelist. Eventually, he settled down to focus on broadcasting and full-time prophesying. As a result, Baxter founded his new prophesying endeavor called End Time Ministries (1991). According to the official website, "The ministry's purpose is to prove that we are now at the end of the era of human government and very near the beginning of the prophesied Kingdom of God."[17] Baxter considers himself to be a part of the Pentecostal movement in the USA and his ministry is very focused on prophecy and, clearly, the end times. In the beginning months of the pandemic, Baxter prophesied that we were in the last days and that pieces of the puzzle were in place for the coming Armageddon. The use of the phrasing in relation to the possibility of the end of the age is significant. The non-committal to a particular date or time for the actual end is important because Baxter had predicted the

[16] Joni Lamb quoted in Carma Hassan, "Christian network television founder and preacher Marcus Lamb, who discouraged vaccinations, dies after being hospitalized for Covid-19," *CNN* (December 2, 2021) https://www.cnn.com/2021/12/01/media/marcus-lamb-covid-death/index.html [accessed 6/27/24].

[17] End Time Ministries, "Who is Irvin Baxter?" End Time Ministries https://www.endtime.com/irvin-baxter/ [accessed 6/27/24].

lead-up to the end of the world several times at this stage. His program was called "End of the Age,"[18] after all. He did think there was a specialness about 2020, but not necessarily for reasons related to the pandemic. In fact, he believed that the pandemic was from an angry God. Why was God angry? "Mr. Baxter had implied [COVID-19] was a punishment from God for the world's sins, which to him included homosexuality, abortion and unmarried couples living together."[19] Baxter believed that the virus was a wake-up call from God and that we might view it as a "privilege,"[20] as it was a far less intense punishment than the coming judgment from God. He concluded that humans could not just continue acting sinful and expect no consequences. Baxter died from complications of COVID-19 on November 3, 2020.

The vaccination debate can go round and round, so I want to focus on the theology behind what both Lamb and Baxter were offering their respective communities. In one sense, you have a broadcaster who is very much in the Word of Faith movement, and on the other hand, you have a broadcaster who leans more into the apocalyptic areas of theology. Both, I would argue, are offering bad theology to their listeners. Lamb stands firmly in the power of the supernatural, above all things. Speaking faithfully is important, and acting faithfully follows suit in this tradition. As a result, if one believes they are going to be healed by the divine, one must believe that with all their being. Part of that belief is not using alternative methods in order to maintain health. According to some, God is all one needs for healing, not the government, or science, or hospitals (I might add). There was a recent report that was published by Texas A and M University about the vaccine and theological beliefs, specifically of those who consider themselves evangelicals (which they acknowledge is a very diverse group). Dr. Heidi Campbell of Texas A and M offered insights into her research on this group. According to Campbell, part of the reason that many evangelicals, and I would argue Word of Faith specifically, do not trust the vaccine is theological. "There's also a general kind of

[18] Neil Genzlinger, "Irvin Baxter, Who Preached the End Was Near, Dies at 75," *New York Times* (November 13, 2020) https://www.nytimes.com/2020/11/13/obituaries/irvin-baxter-dead-covid.html [accessed 6/27/24].

[19] Genzlinger, "Irvin Baxter, Who Preached the End Was Near, Dies at 75."

[20] Yelena Dzhanova, "A Televangelist who referred to the coronavirus as a 'privilege' has died from it," *Business Insider* (November 7, 2020) https://www.businessinsider.com/televangelist-who-called-the-coronavirus-a-privilege-died-from-it-2020-11 [accessed 6/27/24].

theological belief in the sovereignty of God, that He is the one who knows best. So if you get sick, it's because you don't have faith in God and that you're not living a holy life, so God isn't able to protect you."[21]

Lamb adhered to a doctrine that stated that one's health was based on one harnessing the power of God in one's life. It could be argued that one way that humans are able to live in faith in God is through science and through the brains that scientific progress is made. However, this movement inherently is very distrustful of science, and the us versus them of science and religion puts the two at opposing ends. Living according to this doctrine was of the utmost importance to Lamb and his ministries, and he brought people on his show who agreed with the principle of what was being said even if not for the same basic reason. That is, it did not matter why Robert Kennedy Jr. (RFK) disagreed with vaccines as long as he did, because so did Lamb.

Even after Lamb's death, his family maintained the party/doctrine line that was established through Word of Faith. Despite Lamb going to hospital, he still had faith in God healing him. Despite getting oxygen and other scientific care, he still adhered to the beliefs that he had stated on his program about God's power to heal, according to his wife. And then, according to his family, he did not die from some scientific ailment, but instead he died from supernatural means that were trying to silence him. He was unable to combat the evil forces in his state, and so he eventually succumbed to them. He did not give up on God, it is just that the devil became too much and forced his hand (into a hospital).

When we analyze Word of Faith based on my criteria, we see human flourishing is not at the center of the doctrine, even if we just look at the life and death of Marcus Lamb. Naming and claiming, a phrase often used in relation to speaking into existence that which we want in the world, did not work with Lamb. He died of COVID-19, and while his family can construct a narrative of the devil wearing him down, at the end of the day he still died. It is not to say that science is flawless in its approaches, but this does feel like a death that could have been prevented with care in place, especially since he had diabetes.

Word of Faith is not reflective in their theology, you can see this in the response of his family to his death. There is no backtracking on what

[21] Mia Mercer, "Why Evangelicals are Encouraging the Anti-Vaccination Movement," Texas A and M University (May 4, 2021) https://liberalarts.tamu.edu/blog/2021/05/04/why-evangelicals-are-encouraging-the-anti-vaccination-movement/ [accessed 6/27/24].

Lamb said on air, even despite his death. If anything, there is a locking down of what he said and a further explanation of why that theology is true. Despite it being clearly dangerous. There is also isolation in this approach. Theologians like myself look at this theology with sympathy, but ultimately cannot imagine there being no reflection in light of Lamb's death. Word of Faith is largely rejected by the theological community, and it is continuously a theology that gets critiqued according to biblical principles, which it severely lacks. All theology is a construct, as I have claimed, but not all theology is constructed very well. The idea that Word of Faith would consider themselves to be equal to Jesus at any stage, or even to have influence over God is a concept that is not at all widely shared in the Christian community. They are outliers at best, and extremely bad at theology at worst. Lamb died because he believed in his cause. Despite his cause being based on belief, like many others who listened to televangelists like him, he ended up in the grave.

While Baxter had slightly different foci in his ministry, the results were much the same. This time it was not diabetes as an underlying condition, but Baxter's age. That being said, the warning signs were still there that he was not going to make it through this pandemic. Baxter's bad theology is centered on his apocalyptic focus. If you want to read more about bad theology and the inherent issues with end-times theology, you can read my chapter on Jim Jones in *Bad Theology*, but I will also talk about it here. End-times theology is, by its nature, in the moment. The end is near, and the times are short, and your life will be ending soon. As a result, things of this world take a back seat to all things that are otherworldly and immanent. We have seen, especially in cults, the evils that can occur when people blindly follow someone who says the world is ending and none of this earthly stuff matters. It instills in humans a sense that because of the temporal nature of what they are living, they can live or die as they please.

Baxter lived this type of life, perpetually telling his audience that they were not long for this world because Armageddon was upon us. Much like Word of Faith, I would say this is bad theology. The problem with apocalyptic theology is that, as far as we know, no one has been right in their prophecies about the end time. Also, people have done irresponsible, dangerous, and deadly things for people who have said the end is near. There is the illusion of human flourishing within the context of apocalyptic theology, but really it is about the power of the leader who holds the secret to the return of Jesus. Also, the leader holds the power to make people do what they want them to do. This is not human flourishing, but it is human manipulation.

Baxter was careful with his prophesies, which a lot of these types of preachers are not. He used specific language to say that he believed the pieces of the puzzle were coming together in order to lead to Armageddon. A prophecy he could very easily retract, and did, in his history on the airwaves. So, he was giving a false promise to his audience, but making these promises as one with authority. He was able to lure people in that way. I spoke about this on my podcast with Kristy Whaley, *Theology on the Rocks*, and in my research, I have found that there seems to be a desire for some Christians for the whole thing to be over. Not in a death kind of way, but more in a Jesus returns and promises are fulfilled kind of way. This makes sense in our theology, but it also leaves people open for manipulation when religious leaders claim that the end is near and that they know when it is happening.

There is an isolation that comes from this type of prophecy. The relative that I spoke of at the beginning of this book suffered greatly from televangelists who claimed the end was near. They gave money to these folks for their endeavors to prepare the world for the end. What was money, after all, when it was all going to be over soon? This isolated my family member from the rest of the family, as we tried to convince them that they were making a grave error in their financial offerings. I am sure many people succumb to this type of convincing via the TV, especially if they are hoping for Jesus' return to happen in their lifetime.

I have personally experienced the isolation that can occur as a result of this type of programming. In many ways, the televangelists need the person to be isolated. The same as any kind of cult, there is a need for your victims to be in an echo chamber, away from people who might offer alternative opinions. All the while, they are sowing the seeds that those who oppose the prophesies are the "thems." In this case, Baxter not only included those who disagreed with him as thems, but also included a whole host of folks who he believed were sinning. God's wrath, via the virus, was a clear sign of God's anger. Why was God angry? Because of the people in the world who were sexually deviant, according to Baxter's standards. It was clear that *some* people were not doing what they should be doing, and so we all had to suffer from this wake-up call from God. Baxter not only isolates his listeners from those who do not agree with this end-times prophecy but he also separates his listeners from anyone who might be in their lives participating in the fornication that Baxter finds problematic (the LGBTQIA community, people who get abortions, people who live together outside of marriage, etc.). Needless to say, equality is not playing a factor in this theology.

Baxter, in a theological conclusion that many found shocking, stated that the virus was a privilege. It was a privilege because it was a wake-up call from God, and was severe, but was nothing in comparison to the judgment that was to come. I believe this theological twist was a way to comfort those who had had loved ones die from the virus, and I'm sure it was comforting to him in his final days. This suffering was nothing in comparison to that which is on its way, and you better believe that it is on its way, according to Baxter. Get right with God, and live your life right, and await the coming Armageddon, according to Baxter.

Not exactly comforting, right? Maybe not for us, but for his listeners who were in a holding pattern, it meant that the fear of the virus was secondary. This was the initial wrath of God, and maybe it would be a good thing if we got it and died, according to Baxter. It would mean that we miss the wrath that is to come. By constructing a theology whereby the pandemic was not as bad as what everyone was saying, Baxter was able to lull people into a sense of security. Especially, if they had checked off all the boxes for the coming end. There is a major issue with this, of course. If it is one thing people should not do in a pandemic, it is become passive about living life. I'm reminded of the story of William Miller, an apocalyptic storyteller much like Baxter. Miller was a preacher in the nineteenth century, in the early days of the USA. Miller preached that the end of the world was coming soon, and he predicted two dates. The first date came and went and Miller admitted he may have gotten it wrong. He was certain about the second date, however, October 22, 1844. Miller's followers were so convinced of his prediction that they sold all of their land, belongings, and houses. They gave away all of their money, and they climbed on their roofs in order to await the return of Jesus.

Only, October 22, 1844, concluded, and as the morning of October 23 took shape, the Millerites looked around at a world that was the same as the one they had left the night before. It became known as "The Great Disappointment," and Miller was ousted from his position. One Millerite observed: "Our fondest hopes and expectations were blasted, and such a spirit of weeping came over us as I never experienced before … We wept and wept, till the day dawn."[22] I'm reminded of this often when I hear apocalyptic theology. Will one day someone get it right? Maybe. But so far

[22] George Knight, *Millennial Fever and the End of the World* (Boise, ID: Pacific Press, 1993), 218.

it has not been successful, and what it has caused is weeping. Weeping beyond measure. How much weeping did Baxter cause because of his laissez-faire approach to the pandemic, we will never know. It probably would be too much to bear. What we do know is that in the USA there were a million (take out millions and millions!!!) millions and millions people who died as a result of this virus, and there were pastors, called by God to protect God's flock. For many, it felt like it was just another opportunity to practice bad theology and further their own cause.

One thing I do know, "The King will reply, 'Truly I tell you, whatever you did for one of the least of these brothers and sisters of mine, you did for me.'"[23]

That is prophecy enough for me.

[23] New International Version, Matthew 25:40, Bible Gateway https://www.biblegateway.com/passage/?search=Matthew%2025%3A40&version=NIV [accessed 6/28/24].

CHAPTER 8

Conclusion: What Did We Learn?

> But what had he, Rieux, won? No more than the experience of having known plague and remembering it, of having known friendship and remember it, of knowing affection and being destined one day to remember it. So, all a man could win in the conflict between plague and life was knowledge and memories. But Tarrou perhaps, would have called that winning the match.[1]

It is 2024 now, it has been four long years since I sat down and wrote that paper about the pandemic. So much has happened in our world since then, and when I sit down now and try and think about what we have learned, I am reminded of Camus' quote. "So, all a man could win in the conflict between plague and life was knowledge and memories."[2] Knowledge and memories. Did we win those, though? Knowledge, certainly, as our medical professionals raced to find a vaccine to keep us upright in society. As the rest of us adjusted our practices to accommodate a new world (I did finally get my desk in the end). We learned about the world and we learned about ourselves. We learned about how far we could be pushed as a society. Some of us even learned how to make sourdough bread.[3]

[1] Camus, *The Plague*, 291.
[2] Camus, *The Plague*, 291.
[3] Not me, but I did get another cat.

L. Robinson, *Bad Theology in a Time of COVID*,
https://doi.org/10.1007/978-3-031-75294-0_8

As our world became smaller, we realized what a privilege it was to have technology. We learned that Zoom was not necessarily a bad thing because connecting with our relatives was now a thing we longed for beyond belief. We learned that we can connect with people that we have not talked to in a very long time, relatively easily, and we learned that the mute button holds much power. We learned that we had taken a lot of stuff for granted, and that stuff emerged in flaming color when we were utterly denied it. We learned that humans mattered, and we needed to do all we could to protect them. We learned that, as much as it might sting a little, there were essential workers in this world. Workers who did not have the luxury to work from home. And they are what make the world work in real time.

We learned the beauty of being outside. Some of us are outsidey as opposed to outdoorsy, so maybe you did not learn to go on mountain-climbing expeditions, but you do now appreciate a good porch swing. Sunsets come and go, but when they are your main source of entertainment, it is hard not to take notice. We slowed down a little. We were not necessarily happy about it, but we did it anyway. We did it for the good of those around us. My husband has Type 1 Diabetes, and I was a teacher in a classroom every day, so I am certainly happy that people decided to isolate for a while. I worried every moment for him.

And as the weeks turned into months, we learned other things too. We learned that we were not giving up on the things we hold to be important. We would not stop celebrating certain milestones in our lives. They may just have to look different. We held graduations in car processions and weddings in fields. We learned that six feet is the magic number, or maybe it is nine, but we were going to make this work, dang it! And then we also learned disappointment. Those concerts that were lost to the virus. Those Hamilton tickets you waited so long to get. That trip you were going to take that you had saved up for years for. That year of school you will never get back. That deposit on that event that never happened. And there was resentment; of course, there was, but what could we do? We were all sharing in this together.

And then we knew death. That which was someone else's problem became ours very quickly. That first friend who said they had COVID-19 became somewhat of a voyeuristic experiment. And then that first person you knew who died. The first friend. And then the first relative. Maybe you were lucky and this did not happen to you, I certainly pray that was the case. At this point, we were all sharing in collective mourning and collective fear. A sense of dread that this, truly, was never going to end.

In Camus' *The Plague*, this feeling hits the town in the story hard. It is probably one of the most striking scenes. The scene where people have simply stopped hoping that it will end. They have stopped looking at the stats of the dead. They have stopped asking when the town walls might think about being opened. They accepted their status, sure, but they had also accepted that hope was not an emotion that they could rely on anymore. They had resigned themselves that this was the new reality. And there was no end date on this reality. It gets to the point that when the gates are opened, finally, there is not a swarm to escape the town they had been stuck in for years. Instead, the people simply stare at the gate. The world was, as it was, for so long, the idea of hope had completely left their being. The gate opening had lost all of its power over the people.

At its best, theology can offer hope to people. At its worst, it can completely destroy a person. The best of theology is what attracted me to become a minister in the first place, despite the content of this book. There is a hope inherently built into Christianity. The hope that I have spoken about in this book. That this world is not the end of the journey for us. That there is something beyond this world. That we will see our loved ones again. That we will reap the benefits of our good choices and good deeds in a place that is beyond what we know now. That one day, the gate of the city will open, and we will be able to walk right out to our destiny.

The people that I write about in this book were not interested in opening the gate for people. They wanted to close the gate and trap people in a state of fear. This might have been fear of the government, or liberals, or gay people, or even God in some instances. But overwhelmingly, they wanted people to be in fear. Of course, they framed it as liberation, but it was not. Come to church, give money, defy government, do not trust science. Trust us. So, we gained knowledge from them too, but it was from people who absolutely and fundamentally did not have our best interest at heart. They were uniformly selfish in their approach. They wanted us to throw away our knowledge from one source and to take their knowledge as the only truth. Many could argue that the scientists were doing the same thing. Sure, but the scientists I read never asked me to go to a large gathering of people and give them all my money. That part I know to be true, personally.

The other thing we gain in the plague is memories, according to the quote. The interesting thing about memories is they are so easily lost. I am an avid photographer, and part of the reason that I love taking pictures so much is because I love to be able to remember. To look back at nice times, to see the emotions on people's faces. To relive something that was so important to me at the time. It is like feeling that joy all over again. I think it is probably why I like history so much, which will be evident from this book. Unlike most pictures, history is not always joyful to look back on, but no one can say it is not beneficial. But much like any other memory, history too is often lost so easily, and it was this overwhelming feeling that pervaded my writing of this text.

History is so enticing for an educator because I truly think that if I can just show someone what it was like back then, then it will be different in the future. As I began to look up the theological reactions to pandemics throughout history, I was torn apart. Even from the early church, you have the hopelessness of the Stoics, Epicureans, and Platonists who remind me so intensely of these apocalyptic preachers during COVID-19. None of it matters, so we might as well just fit in and wait it out. We are destined for a different world, so this one really does not matter.

When looking at the Catholic church in the Black Death, I was left with a feeling of déjà vu. The plague is not a result of anything earthly but is simply God's wrath upon society. The reasons for God's wrath is because the world has abandoned God for other things. This reads a lot like a sermon from Drollinger, but it is not. Over and over in the COVID-19 pandemic, we hear about God's wrath being the root cause of the suffering that is taking place. One minister goes so far as to say that the virus is God. All of this sounds very medieval, and for good reason, it is. We are still selling holy trinkets to protect us from bad things, but instead of medals of St. Roch, we are selling holy handkerchiefs and over-hyped hand sanitizer at 80 dollars a pop.

When we compare the history of pandemics in this text to that of our current day, we begin to see that not much has changed. Memories are tough because they are so easily lost. We somehow lost these memories despite the extensive history. Heck, we might have lost the memories of people saying HIV/AIDS was the wrath of God against people who were seen by some in the church as being sexually deviant. That was in my life time, and yet here we are again as if this is a new argument about COVID-19. The scary alternative is that we do remember, but we just think it to be true, so the story gets repeated. Memories are tough because they are so easily lost, but some memories are tough because they are not easily lost.

So, when I reflect on my writing, and I think about what we have learned, I am sometimes at a loss. When I began this conclusion, I just sat and stared at my notes. What had we learned? I could be pessimistic here, but I hope that I have gotten that out of the way with my history rant. Knowledge can be manipulated and memories can be lost, and that is two terrible outcomes of traumatic situations like the one that we have been in for the past four years. What I can leave you with is what I hope we have learned from our experiences.

I hope that we have learned how to spot bad theology a mile away. This is my second book on this topic, and while I do think I am better at spotting bad theology out in the wild-I do think that I can hone my skill a bit better. I am an awfully big fan of people generally speaking, and this can sometimes be a disadvantage in the naming and shaming aspect. I hope as well that we have learned how to discuss bad and good theology with people in a way that is productive and meaningful. Something else that we lost in the pandemic was the ability to disagree. Suddenly disagreements about various things could lead to the breakup of a family. I sincerely hope that this book, and the previous one, can lead to good conversations between people who may disagree with one another on one of the topics discussed. I miss conversations that end with a chuckle and a nod and a knowledge that no one is changing anyone's mind here, but there is still deep love and respect.

I hope that we are able to see that theology is a social construct, and that construct can work for good or ill. There is 0% of me that agrees that the virus was a result of God's wrath. Though I'll wait to ask God about that one to confirm (hopefully it will be a few years yet). The importance of knowing that mine, yours, and their theology is constructed is not to send the world into mass confusion. It is to be able to see the world as simultaneously searching for God actively, and also being chained to your own brain in the process. A brain that was developed in a time and a place. Full of bias and inconsistencies. This should be a space of mercy for people. Also, a space of discernment. Mercy that you or I may not have Kaufman's reality God, and that is ok. Also, that if you claim to have a piece of reality God, I have a means of evaluating that.

In a conference recently, a student said, "The criteria is very much based on the language of someone who is xyz." They were absolutely correct in their assessment of my xyzs. I said, certainly, I am also incredibly guilty of constructing my own theological standards. But the difference between what some of these people doing bad theology are saying and what I am saying is that I *know* that I am constructing it. I am also not asking anyone else to adhere to what I am saying. They can accept or reject it or accept parts and reject others. This is not a luxury that is offered in many of the examples that I gave in the book. It is also not a theological exercise that is always embraced in historical theology; see the story about Karl Barth in the book. I can't always promise much, but I do promise I will not shout NO! at you at a conference for disagreeing with me.

I hope that we can take a look at our own history and evaluate what theological ideas are learned and evaluate those that have been ingrained in the very soul of our nation through time. There are a few theological claims that I would say need to go directly in the bin, but certainly prosperity gospel would be one of them. I have not found much worth in this theological conclusion, except for maybe positive thinking as a good exercise. It has done far more harm to people that I know, and ones I do not, than it has helped. It is not to say that good theology is always self-serving, far from it, but this theology has no real grounding in, well, anything. It is bad theology, and it is damaging theology, and its biblical claims are strenuous at best. The high anthropological ideas of both prosperity and the New Thought movement are dangerous in the hands of the wrong people. For reference to the wrong people, see the last two chapters. If I was in charge of the moon door, Game of Thrones reference two, I would be pulling the hatch on that one.

In contrast, premillennialism is a theology that is difficult to send down the drain. It is a part of the very core of our hope as Christians that Jesus will return one day. We just have not quite figured out the order in which it will happen, what else will happen at the time, or when exactly it all might happen. Inherently, I do not see an issue with contemplating such things. That being said, I do see a severe difference in thinking about those things and living your life exclusively on the basis of those things. There is a danger in Christians not having something to lose on this earth. We are here for a relatively short amount of time, but the idea that we would not feel connected to the earth or those on it is a terrifying thought. While we can certainly hope for future promises, I do not think we should metaphorically sell all our belongings and climb on a roof anytime soon. We see the dangers of that pretty clearly when faced with a global pandemic.

Also, these apocalyptic theologies are rife for manipulation. When a group of people have no fear of earthly consequences, then you can get them to do your bidding pretty easily. If there is no worth seen in the here and now, then it is very easy indeed to discredit any and all worries that the current life holds. Focus the mind on that which is coming soon, and that which is happening right now can easily be ignored.

And those pesky politicians and their partisanship, what do we do with them? In many ways, this is a subject for Political Studies PhDs to handle, but I do have some thoughts here from a theological perspective. Much like the quote in the beginning of my book, power only resides where people believe it resides. Power is a construct, and we are the ones who construct it. We create superheroes and we create politicians, but they are not one and the same, despite what they might have you believe. Their power comes from the people who believe in what they do and say. Increasingly, their power comes from them pitting people against one another. Creating a system of us versus them, not reflecting on their actions, isolating their followers, creating an echo chamber of like-minded individuals, and not focusing on equality or justice (unless it serves them). This is beginning to sound kind of familiar…

We also cannot let them tear us apart through using our beliefs and passions against us. We are allowed to think differently from our loved ones and still remain loved ones. Diversity is never a bad thing. Do I want my candidate to win? Of course, I do, but I also know that candidates should not be causing families to split apart. Or people to walk away from the things they love dearly. Or violence or chaos to occur in their name. They only have power because we give them power, so it may be about time we remind them that they serve the entire community, not just the "us."

Finally, those church leaders and televangelists, what do I hope in that regard? Other than opening back up that moon door I spoke about before, there needs to be a healthy dose of reckoning for some of these people. And honestly, I am not so egotistical to think the reckoning should come from me, nor do I think it would have much effect for that matter. I hope that churches where the minister is operating similar to the way I described will hold their leaders accountable. If you are in a church where you do not feel comfortable with the rhetoric that is being preached or taught, you are allowed to say something. One of the saddest things I read on this topic, and that is saying a lot, was in MacArthur's church during COVID-19. The congregants felt too scared to report that they were getting sick for fear of retribution. Not from MacArthur, but from their fellow churchgoers. Power only resides where people believe it resides, and if we see this type of thing happening in the church, there is a change that needs to take place. We cannot let non-theological culture wars being wielded by wannabe theologians and politicians, tear us apart in the church. If your minister sounds more like a politician than a person of God, it might be time to remind them of their job description.

That being said, in regard to the established church, I do not believe that there should be external interference in the day-to-day workings. This plays too much into a leader who is already sowing the seeds of confusion and paranoia about outside sources. Instead, I do feel as though there is a need for internal audits. No one minister or leader should ever have complete control over a church. The church has always been a collection of believers. When there is a cult of personality over one individual in the church, the dynamics have shifted significantly in this regard. It makes it super difficult for change to occur, so it is important to recognize the shift as it is occurring. We must be as wise as serpents, as the good book says.

All that aside, this is not the same case with the televangelists. The FCC used to be able to regulate these stations based on the interest of the common good. This does not seem to be the case any longer, and it is high time for that to change. I know that this will be a difficult task based on the mass followings that a lot of these leaders have, but they are ruining people's lives across the nation. It is one thing to have a pastor in a church preach a message you do not agree with, but these televangelists are preying on vulnerable people with no checks and balances whatsoever. There are no deacons that reel them in, or members of the congregation that tell them that they took things too far. There is no transparent budgetary committee that tells them they've exceeded their donation goal, but based on their jail time that might not be a bad idea for them. These people are frauds, they are manipulative, they exemplify bad theology, and they need to be off the airwaves or heavily regulated. Sermon complete.

A final, and super heartfelt, hope is that this entire exercise strengthens your faith. That it does not send you into a tailspin of what it all means, but it helps you to equip yourself to try and fight against these small people with big shadows. I am a part of the Christian community, and I have zero interest in watching it crumble around me. I am also an academic theologian who had to sit by and watch as these articles, albeit few and far between, make my religion look ridiculous, on repeat. It was truly a crazy time to be alive, and we will be telling the stories about COVID-19 for the rest of our lives.

But remember, the danger in memories is that they are so easily lost. We must not lose the feeling we had when we read about Jim Bakker and his silver solution, or about John MacArthur and his condemnation of entire communities of people. We must not forget our memories of when Tony Spell promised elderly people they would be saved from COVID-19 by gathering in large groups. We must not forget the way we watched people like Marcus Lamb say that hospitals were not helpful for the general public, while he himself passed away in one. We must not believe that COVID-19 was God's wrath. God's wrath did not cause over one million Americans to die right before our eyes. God's people spread the virus, but God's people also brought us back from the brink and saved us from that virus. We must never forget that.

Power resides where we believe it resides. It's a trick. A shadow on the wall. And for far too long we have let far too many very small people cast too big of a shadow on our world. I hope that we change that really soon. I'll start, so there once was this man named Jerry Falwell, Jr...

What would your introduction look like?

> Saruman believes that it is only great power that can hold evil in check, but that is not what I found. I found it is the small things, every day deeds of ordinary folk that keeps the darkness at bay. Simple acts of kindness and love.
>
> -Gandalf, *Lord of the Rings*

Index[1]

[1] Note: Page numbers followed by 'n' refer to notes.

L. Robinson, *Bad Theology in a Time of COVID*,
https://doi.org/10.1007/978-3-031-75294-0

SPRINGER NATURE

GPSR Compliance

The European Union's (EU) General Product Safety Regulation (GPSR) is a set of rules that requires consumer products to be safe and our obligations to ensure this.

If you have any concerns about our products, you can contact us on ProductSafety@springernature.com

In case Publisher is established outside the EU, the EU authorized representative is:

Springer Nature Customer Service Center GmbH
Europaplatz 3
69115 Heidelberg, Germany

The manufacturer's authorised representative in the EU is Springer Nature Customer Service Centre GmbH, Europaplatz 3, 69115 Heidelberg, Germany. If you have any concerns regarding our products, please contact ProductSafety@springernature.com

Printed and bound by CPI Group (UK) Ltd, Croydon, CR0 4YY
30/09/2026
02225514-0009